A Blueprint for
Better Health

A Blueprint for Better Health

A dietary guide to counteract diseases

Louis S. de Villiers
B.Sc., M.B. Ch.B., M.Med. (Path.)

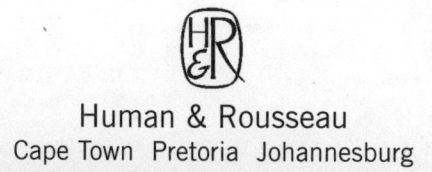

Human & Rousseau
Cape Town Pretoria Johannesburg

Copyright © 1998 by Louis S. de Villiers
Published by Human & Rousseau (Pty) Ltd
State House, 3-9 Rose Street, Cape Town
Cover design by Chérie Collins
Typography by Robert Meas
Typeset in 10.5 on 12.5 pt Trade Gothic by Human & Rousseau
Printed and bound by National Book Printers
Drukkery Street, Goodwood, Western Cape

ISBN 0 7981 3748 7

No part of this book may be reproduced or transmitted in any form
or by any means, electronic or mechanical or by photocopying,
recording or microfilming, or stored in any retrieval system,
without the written permission of the publisher

FOREWORD

Many books and journal articles have been published on the relation between diet and chronic diseases of lifestyle. Yet few are as stimulating, as provocative, as Professor Louis de Villiers's *A Blueprint for Better Health*. In a book that will appeal to both the medical professional and the layman, Professor De Villiers shifts the emphasis from a low-fat to a high micronutrient diet in the prevention of lifestyle diseases that continue to plague industrialised communities. Although *A Blueprint for Better Health* focuses on the beneficial effects of a diet rich in fibre and micronutrients in the prevention of coronary heart disease, the book also contains valuable information on the role of diet in hypertension, diabetes, obesity and osteoporosis.

A Blueprint for Better Health emphasises the role of homocysteine in vascular disease. Professor De Villiers was in fact one of the few medical specialists who, as far back as 1982, had the foresight to recognise that an elevated blood homocysteine concentration may be a causative factor of coronary heart disease. In 1982 the scientific information on blood homocysteine levels was limited (with only 15 papers published in the medical literature during that year) and Professor De Villiers was scorned for his ideas, which were considered radical and irresponsible. Yet, today, 16 years later, even the staunchest opponents of De Villiers's ideas have to acknowledge that homocysteine is widely recognised as a risk factor for premature cardiovascular diseases. It is for this reason that Professor De Villiers's book is so timely. Although the scientific literature is abuzz with the possible adverse effects of elevated blood homocysteine concentrations (374 papers dealing with the subject published in 1997), few people on the street have ever heard about homocysteine. *A Blueprint for Better Health* does not only describe the role of homocysteine in cardiovascular disease, but gives practical dietary guidelines to control this risk factor.

A Blueprint for Better Health is not only concerned with pathophysiological principles, but it is in fact a very practical book that will lead the reader step by step to choose an appropriate micronutrient rich diet. Professor De Villiers makes it perfectly clear that a high micronutrient diet is not simply achieved by adding a multivitamin supplement to your diet. In his characteristic humorous way he discounts various objections raised against the high micronutrient diet. He warns against an overemphasis on lipid lowering diets and drugs and he sensitises the reader to the many commercial interests confusing the field of preventive medicine. De Villiers recognises, however, that diet is only one part of a healthy lifestyle. The book therefore also contains valuable information on how to stop smoking, to moderate alcohol intake, to relax and to ensure sufficient physical exercise.

Professor De Villiers's ideas on the interaction between genetics and diet are thought provoking. Again, we are faced with a fascinating hypothesis, but (still) little evidence. Nevertheless, who knows, 16 years onwards . . .

I heartily recommend reading this book. The lifestyle principles highlighted in this book are well worth pursuing.

Prof Job Ubbink
Professor: Department of Chemical Pathology
University of Pretoria

CONTENTS

Acknowledgements   9
Introduction   11
Explanation and Interpretation of References   15
Glossary of Terms   17

1. Genetics: The Human Computer   19
2. Micronutrients: Small Things and Big Problems   30
3. The Amazing World of Fatty Acids   39
4. Coronary Heart Disease: Fact or Fiction   58
5. A Complete Theory on Atherosclerosis   88
6. Lifestyle   105
7. The Genetic Micronutrient Diet   113
8. The Other Greater Metabolic Diseases   133
9. A Diet for Overweight   156
10. Other and Lesser Modern Diseases   163
11. In Conclusion   177

Appendixes   179
Index   185

ACKNOWLEDGEMENTS

This book is my third on the subject, following on *Your Heart: The Unrefined Facts*, of which I was chief contributing author, and *You and Your Diet: Nature's Computer*, of which I was sole author. Appropriate acknowledgements were made in both publications, but I must again mention several distinguished colleagues.

Professor Hayward Vermaak, my successor in my former department at Pretoria University, lent his continued support, as did Professor Job Ubbink, who kept me informed of the latest developments regarding homocysteine. I was encouraged by the interest shown by two consecutive rectors of the University, Professor Danie Joubert (since deceased) and Professor Flip Smit. Three previous heads of the Department of Internal Medicine, Professors Hennie Snyman, Barney Ziady and Boet Kloppers, never wavered in showing interest in the new line of thought I was adopting. Like Danie Joubert all three have, alas, died and are sorely missed – particularly Boet Kloppers, a good friend whose telephonic communications from afar were much appreciated.

My heartfelt thanks are due, too, to the commanding officer and his staff of No 2 Military Hospital, Wynberg, who allowed me to apply the principles of treatment described in this book in ideal circumstances where patients were seen on a regular ongoing basis, returning monthly for further treatment. I owe a debt of gratitude to these patients for the enthusiasm with which they followed my recommendations.

I am happy to take this opportunity of thanking several distinguished world leaders in medicine with whom I have corresponded, and for whose advice I have always been grateful (even when I have disagreed with it). They include Professor Michael Oliver of Edinburgh and London, Dr Michael DeBakey of the USA (who treated President Yeltsin in Moscow), Professor Michael Horrobin of Efamol fame, Professor Walter Willett of Harvard Medical School, and American nutritionists Dr Mildred Seelig and Dr Mary Enig.

Last, but very far from least, I salute my wife, Annamarie, who, at the age of forty-five and a mother of seven children (hers, mine and ours), abandoned a successful career as a psychologist and teacher to study medicine, claiming our research as her inspiration for taking this step. Despite having become a busy general practitioner, she was on hand at all times to encourage, support and advise me.

Louis S. de Villiers
Hermanus, 1998

INTRODUCTION

With the resources of constantly developing technology, ongoing research in every area of medical science, and an expanding armoury of drugs and advanced surgical procedures, medicine has come a long way since the days of its ancient Greek founding father, Hippocrates.

Nonetheless, miraculous cures for the two most prevalent killer diseases of the late 20th century, coronary heart disease and cancer, have yet to be found. All medical students, at some idealistic stage of their studies, dream of discovering such cures while, at the same time, we have all by and large come to believe that heart attacks, cancer, high blood pressure, diabetes and other debilitating and sometimes fatal illnesses are inevitable facts of later life about which little can be done.

There is little doubt that people nowadays expect and, indeed, demand more information about illness than ever before, and it is primarily for the concerned and interested layman who wishes to know more than the popular media and hospital soap operas provide, that this book has been written. I must, however, ask the lay reader to bear with me and have the patience to surmount or ignore the several passages in the text which are too technical or scientific for his purpose. I have felt it incumbent on myself to provide scientific facts in support of my views in order to deflect the criticism of those trained experts whose views may differ from my own.

Basically, the intention of the book is to acquaint the reader with the principles of micronutrients and genetics, and so enable him or her to pursue health through diet and to counteract the lurking dangers of heart, cancer and other diseases.

Put simply, micronutrients are the vitamins and minerals necessary for the proper functioning of the body while genetics, in this context, refer to the dietary conditioning of individuals based upon their racial and geographical heredity. Over the years, we medical scientists have diligently followed each new argument pointing out the dangers of various fats and fatty acids, cholesterol, triglycerides and so forth, and observed recommendations such as substituting margarine for butter, only to be confounded by the fact that, despite adjustments in diet, little dent was made in the incidence of heart attacks, cancer and other illnesses.

The sceptics were quick to point out that the now forbidden foods were eaten in abundance a few generations back, yet people used to live to a ripe old age free from heart attacks. The proposal that previous generations were free from stress and took more exercise didn't, somehow, seem to address the problem. Whichever way one looked at it, all research showed that the majority of serious diseases of the late 20th century have a history of a hundred years or less. Somewhere there had to be an answer. Perhaps we were looking too deep? As Elbert Hubbard (1856-1915), the American author noted for his vigorous, epigrammatic style, said, "Little minds are interested in the extraordinary; grand minds in the ordinary."

In 1982, my own thoughts on dietary process and diseases underwent a change when I first heard about the substance homocysteine. It was postulated that increased levels of homocysteine in the blood led to atherosclerosis, the forerunner to heart attacks, and that this dangerous increase was caused by a dietary loss of vitamin B6. But what caused the loss of vitamin B6? In their book, *Beyond Cholesterol. Vitamin B6, Arteriosclerosis, and Your Heart*, American physiologists E.R. Gruberg and S.A. Raymond pointed to the refining of food, which began with the introduction of roller mills in 1880.

Much excited by this, we embarked on a thorough programme of reading and research, scouring medical literature both old and new. We made the exciting discovery that homocysteine and vitamin B6 were merely cogs in the complex wheel of medical science, turning in a world of vitamins and minerals closely associated with, and yet independent of, human genes that had been developing over thousands of years.

Everything fitted neatly into a pattern which closely resembled a computer – well organised and well orchestrated, but with one essential difference: the computer's programme could not be readily changed or even hurried along. Not for a thousand years.

Before attacking the problems, we spent two years reading, thinking, doubting and searching (a process that continues) before beginning to evolve logical solutions to health problems which, though still scorned by the super-specialist, are increasingly accepted by the nutritionist and by the man in the street. No longer are vitamins regarded only as antidotes to scurvy. They are at the forefront in the battle against our most common killer diseases and, with their historic allies, the minerals, form the cornerstone of modern scientific therapeutics.

Some might regard this book as advocating "alternative" medicine. I would suggest that it is indeed alternative – alternative to some seventy years of disappointing and inconclusive treatment, alternative to commercially driven therapeutics. All I can say is that, after five years in general medical practice and thirty-one years as head of an academic chemical pathology laboratory in Pretoria, where I developed a growing interest in clinical nutrition, I returned to general practice to apply the principles of micronutrient and genetic human computerisation. The results have been most gratifying. A stint at a squatter town day hospital and fifteen months at the No 2 Military Hospital, both in Cape Town, more than strengthened my belief in these principles as a simple, inexpensive and effective therapy which I continue to administer.

The American writer and philosopher Ralph Waldo Emerson (1803-1882) said, "The end of the human race will be that it will eventually die of civilisation." That was a hundred years ago; we haven't much time left. Civilisation has brought us food refining, canning, refrigeration and additives, all of which have denuded our diets of necessary micronutrients, and has seen the rise of commercial interests which dictate health "solutions" that are sometimes more dangerous than the condition they seek to correct. We are drowning in ill-considered myths, misinformation and contradictory research with further adverse effects on our wellbeing.

In this book, I have sought to give the reader a history of genetic origins and development and to explain how vitamins and minerals, or the lack of same, affect the enzymes in the body to produce either healthy functioning, or faulty functioning leading to heart attacks and other illness.

I have sought, too, to explain the effect of modern food techniques on diet and the negative results of commercial interests which have too often dictated opinion. My thesis is supported by documented research from which I have quoted, and I've taken care to name all sources – tedious, perhaps, but necessary in the interests of truth.

I urge the reader to note the logic of my arguments and to apply the principles of a micronutrient diet to his or her own life – a life which, far from banning butter, meat and milk, encourages the sensible enjoyment of these foods. Pharmaceutical companies who make cholesterol-lowering drugs and antihypertensives, cardiac surgeons, the vegetable-oil industries and the food manufacturers will not be overjoyed by these arguments, but they have had their day. It is now time for the poor suffering patients to have theirs.

EXPLANATION AND INTERPRETATION OF REFERENCES

The internationally recognised method of publishing references is as follows. First the accepted abbreviation of the journal in which the publication appears, followed immediately by the year of publication, then a semicolon followed by the number of the volume; then a colon followed by the page numbers from start to finish of the article. For example: (*NEJM* 1996; 234: 546-52): *New England Journal of Medicine* 1996; Volume 234: pages 546 to 552. *Med J* always means Medical journal.

Recognised abbreviations of leading medical journals:
    BMJ: British Medical Journal
    Lancet: No abbreviation
    JAMA: Journal of the American Medical Association
    Am J Clin Nutr: American Journal of Clinical Nutrition
    Am J Epid: American Journal of Epidemiology
    Ann Int Med: Annals of Internal Medicine
    Ann Rheum Dis: Annals of Rheumatic Diseases
    Arch Int Med: Archives of Internal Medicine
    Fortschr Med: Fortschrift Medicin
    Med Hypothesis: Medical Hypothesis
    JAOCS: Journal of American Oil Company Standards
    J Am Coll Cardiology: Journal of the American College of Cardiology
    J Med Genetics: Journal of Medical Genetics
    J Royal Coll Physic: Journal of the Royal College of Physicians
    Postgrad Med J: Postgraduate Medical Journal

GLOSSARY OF TERMS

apoprotein: the protein part which binds to lipids (fats)
amino acids: the basic structure of proteins
atherosclerosis: an irregular thickening of the inner layers of arteries
auto-immune disease: one in which antibodies formed in the body are directed against the organ or structure that forms it
carbohydrates: sugars, starches or glycogen, containing a precise empirical formula $(CH2O)n$
CHD (coronary heart disease): narrowing of the blood vessels of the heart due to atherosclerosis, frequently the forerunner of heart attacks
cisfatty acids: a fatty acid where the two carbon atoms of an unsaturated (double) bond are in the same direction in space; this is usually the natural form
co-factors: essential factors which stimulate enzymes, invariably micronutrients
complex carbohydrates: large molecules (in contrast to sugar's small molecules) containing mainly starches
conventional treatment: the most commonly used present treatment
DNA (deoxyribonucleic acid): the structure in all cells containing genetic information in chromosomes
dominant hereditary disease: a hereditary disease in which symptoms are present even when inherited from one parent
EFA (essential fatty acids): two fatty acids, linoleic and alpha-linolenic acid, mainly of dietary origin
endothelium: the inner layer of cells lining the blood vessels
fatty acids: a basic structure of lipids (fats), which binds to other molecules, such as glycerol and apoproteins
genetic: hereditary
HDL-cholesterol (high density lipoprotein cholesterol): mainly formed in the peripheral tissue and organs and carried back to the liver
HLA (human lymphocytic antigen): proteins on the surface of all body cells containing nuclei, that allow the body to recognise and reject foreign tissue; they are closely associated with certain diseases

homozygote: a person who inherits the same disease from both parents
incidence: the number of cases affected per 100 000 of the population
LDL-cholesterol (low density lipoprotein cholesterol): mainly formed in the liver and transported to the organs and tissues of the body
lipoproteins: combination of lipids with proteins
macronutrients: nutrients with relatively large molecules, either proteins, carbohydrates or fats
metabolism: the biochemical reactions in the body needed for normal final products
metabolic disease: a disease in which the metabolism of the body is abnormal or decreased
micronutrients: nutrients with small molecules, either vitamins or minerals, acting mainly as co-factors to enzymes
mutation: a hereditary change in a cell produced by a spontaneous or stimulated alteration of DNA
nutrient: a substance providing nourishment
optimal: at the most favourable concentration
placebo: a compound used in studies which looks and tastes similar to the drug under investigation, but has no metabolic effect; used in the "control group"
polymorphism: more than one form
proteins: chemical structures containing nitrogen (N), the main building stones of the body
PUFA (poly-unsaturated fatty acids): fatty acids which have more than one unsaturated double bond
receptor system: the presence of receptors on cells which allow only specific unique molecules to become attached
supplementation: substances added over and above the diet
transfatty acids: fatty acids in which the two carbon atoms of an unsaturated (double) bond are in the opposite (trans) direction in space, usually an unnatural compound

CHAPTER 1

GENETICS: THE HUMAN COMPUTER

Man is still the most extraordinary computer of all.
JOHN F. KENNEDY, 21 MAY 1963

Introduction

The above words, uttered by a great statesman, were prophetic. Growing evidence exists that the human body is indeed like a sophisticated computer, divinely designed, meticulously programmed, and controlled by genetics and environment.

Many computer functions were old hat to man long before the computer age and its jargon. Man's offspring (back-ups), his foods (insert modes), his metabolism (random-access memory), his biochemical receptors (data bases) were established at least a thousand years ago, man's magical millennium. Leading geneticists agree that it takes approximately a thousand years for man's genetic metabolism to achieve harmony with the diet available to him which, in its turn, is determined by climate. The key concept here is genetic metabolism, because this implies a genetic diet, which is the crucial issue explored in this book.

Over thousands of years different climates and the resultant foodstuffs led to the evolution of at least thirteen genetic races. Nature thus laid the foundations, the programmes were written and the human computer is equipped to be "in sync" with his environment. It is up to man, the Creature of Reason, to make the right choices for healthiness and happiness.

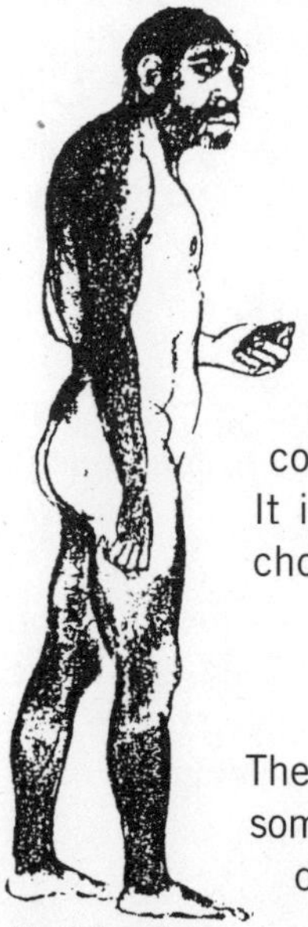

The Appearance of Man

The first four-legged creature that could walk erect appeared some 1.8 million years ago, *Homo erectus* (Fig 1.1). His descendents discovered fire, probably caused by lightning, perhaps some 500 000 years ago, thereby allowing them to eat softer braised meat. It has been concluded that this chewing of softer meat enhanced the more ele-

Fig 1.1.
Homo erectus.

gant shape of his chin, as compared to that of his less intelligent distant cousins, still grinding away at raw meat.

Even at this period differences in diet played a role in the bodily development of man, the heavy robust type following a mainly vegetarian diet, while the more graceful and slender forms developed from a combined meat-vegetable diet.

Modern man, *Homo sapiens*, appeared less than 100 000 years ago. However, it was when man discovered that animals such as horses, cattle, sheep and goats could be domesticated, and that certain seed-bearing plants could be cultivated, that the most dramatic advance in civilisation occurred. This was barely 10 000 years ago, although some authorities cite some late archaeological discoveries to claim that in certain areas of the world it could have been as long as 23 000 years ago (*Whittaker's Almanac*, 1994, p. 1186). Domestication, therefore, brought about a profound change in man's eating habits and lifestyle.

The Bible and Evolution

Professor Jerry Aikowa, Professor of Medicine at the University of Colorado, states in his book *Magnesium: Its Biological Significance*, 1981, that there is a clear correlation between evolutionary events since the beginning of the earth, and those described in The Book of Genesis. Only the length and distribution of time differs.

Domestication during the Last 10 000 Years

Archaeologists and ecologists have obtained evidence that three primary centres of civilisation developed, which in time spread to other areas in the world (Fig 1.2).

These three regions were:

1. The Middle East or Fertile Crescent which extended from Egypt, through South West Asia to the Persian Gulf some 10 000 years ago. Here early farmers grew wheat, barley, lentils and peas. Farming spread to the Nile Valley some 6 500 years ago with wheat, sorghum and barley being the main crops. About 3 500 years ago farming had spread to Abyssinia, with millet and sorghum as the main crops. It is important to stress that sorghum became the staple food of the African.

2. Central America (Southern Mexico, Guatemala, Honduras) became another pioneer farming centre some 7 500 years ago, producing maize,

GENETICS: THE HUMAN COMPUTER • 21

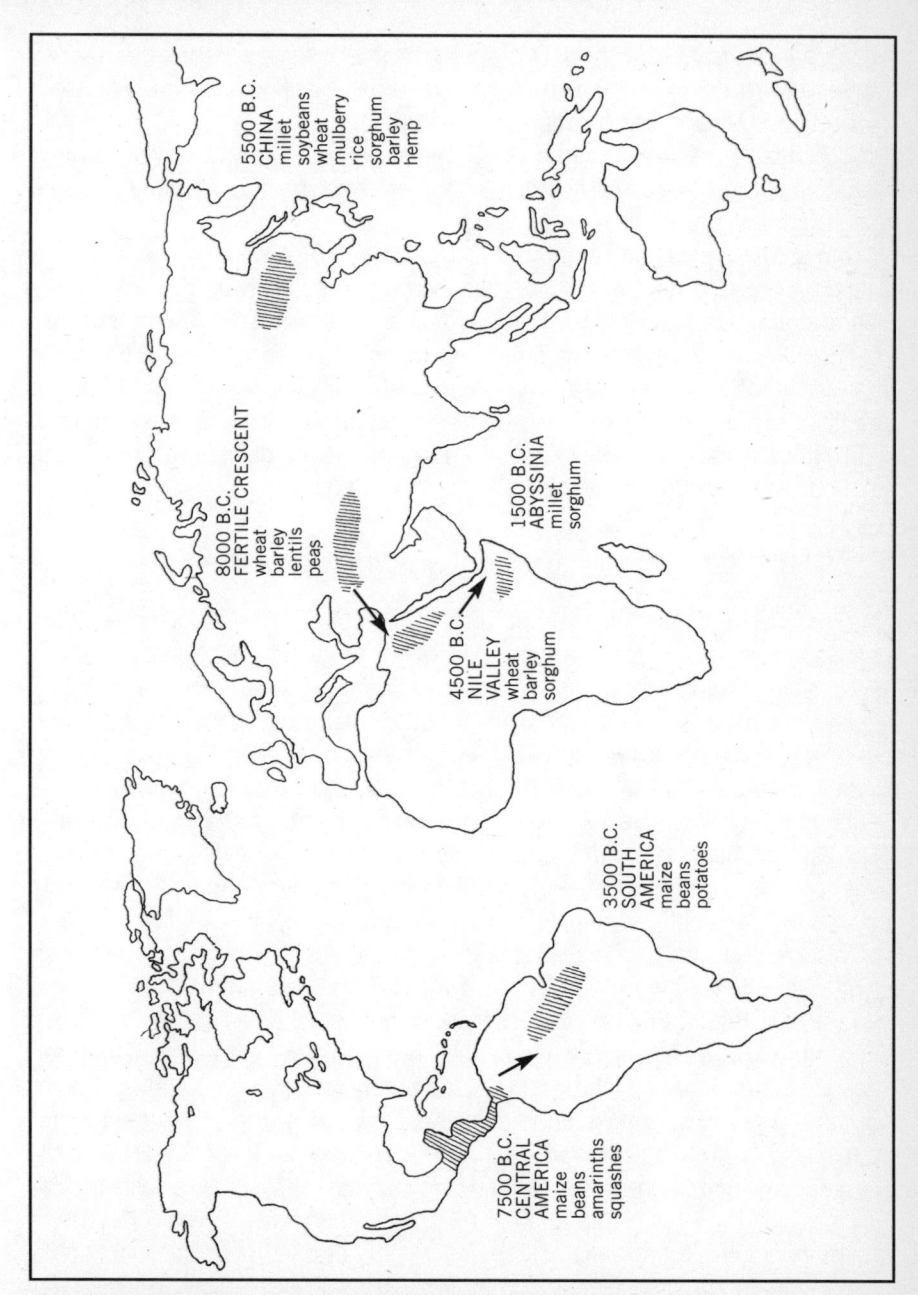

Fig 1.2. The three primary centres of civilisation with later spread to other areas, including the main food crops initiated in those areas.

beans and squashes. Only 4 000 years later did farming spread to South America, with the main crops being maize, alpaca, beans and potatoes. Note that originally maize was primarily an American product.

3. North China where, some 5 500 years ago, the third original farming development occurred, with crops of millet, soya beans, wheat, mulberry, rice, sorghum, barley and hemp.

It must, however, be remembered that man's diet was not restricted to vegetarian foodstuffs (which included certain fruits, berries and roots long before grains were available). He also had access to animal foods, such as meat, milk, butter, eggs, fish and shell foods. It is reasonable to conclude that all the above-mentioned foods were available in varying amounts to the primitive civilisations. Meat, fish and shell foods were available before general domestication, but milk, butter and eggs mainly date from domestication 10 000 to 5 000 years ago.

Nature's and Man's Programmer

It is reasonable to conclude that nature's – particularly man's – dietary genetic "programmer" came into optimum production with the advent of domestication. A new chapter in programming could now be perfected. Furthermore, man's diet would remain reasonably constant for the next five to ten thousand years, and his "computers" could now be perfected and reinforced.

But, man and civilisation were on the move, thanks to whatever primitive communication and travel existed in those times, and new settlements appeared as a result of these wanderings. There, human numbers increased through propagation, leading to the emergence of different races. Certain individual aspects of diets varied, and the ever-present human computer complied with the differing requirements of newly available local foods. A thousand years, however, would prove necessary to establish its own dominant programme.

In 1964 Dr W.C. Boyd and his co-workers published an article in *Taxonomic Biochemistry and Serology*, wherein they described the existence of thirteen separate genetic races in the world, based purely on genetic red-cell groups or antigens. They were the Amerindians, the Laplanders, the North-West Europeans, the Central-East Europeans, the Mediterraneans, the Early Europeans, the Africans, the Indo-Dravidians, the Sino-Japanese, the Indonesians, the Melanesians, the Polynesians and the Australian Aborigines. As expected, these groups coincided with the major race groups in the world, as well as with smaller race groups in more isolated communities.

Boyd's genetic races were divided into five main groups. The early American group, known as the Amerindians, included the Red Indians. In the Pacific Ocean four subgroups are recognised, largely based upon the then relatively isolated island communities of Indonesians, Polynesians, Melanesians and Australian Aborigines. Two groups are recognised in the East, Indo-Dravidian and Asian or Sino-Japanese. In Africa only one group is identified. Significantly, the European group consists of no less than five subgroups, North-Western, East-Central, early Europeans, Mediterranean and the Laplanders. Possibly more groups may exist, e.g. Masai and Pygmies.

The significance of this is that, to promote good health among all, man now has at least thirteen specific genetic diets, programmed over approximately a thousand years, for thirteen corresponding genetic races. These genetic changes could affect either a chemical compound or a relevant enzyme or a relevant receptor. Numerous examples of these facts will be demonstrated later in the text.

Examples of Nonprogrammed Foods

One of the most significant changes has been an increase in polyunsaturated fatty acids (PUFAs). From 1909-1913 the percentage of linoleic acid, the most common PUFA in man, in the USA diet was 2.7% of total dietary energy. This was mainly derived from animal fats. By 1980 the figure had risen to 6.4%, now largely from vegetable fats. But the human body had been programmed for at least a thousand years to metabolise only approximately 2.7% (Krause and Mahon, *Food, Nutrition and Diet Therapy*, 7th Edit. 1984, p 49). The body had too few receptors for these increased PUFAs, and numerous publications in leading medical journals now warn against this increase, citing cases of cancer (animal experiments), allergies and skin diseases.

The same principle applies to margarine. Vegetable oils are converted to solid fats by hydrogenation, i.e. two hydrogen atoms are added to an unsaturated carbon atom at a very high temperature (see Fig 1.3). This is how margarines are produced. But the body has no receptors for these foreign newly formed structures, which now float around the body as foreign substances, causing many problems. See later for further discussion.

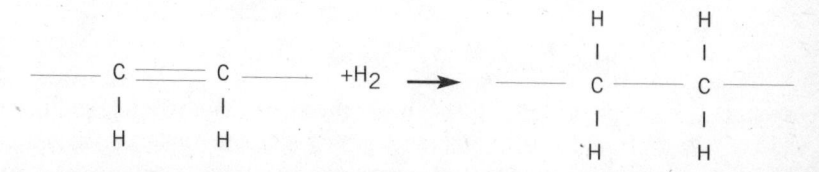

$$\begin{array}{c}\\ -C=C- \\ | \quad\ \ | \\ H \quad\ H\end{array} \quad +H_2 \longrightarrow \quad \begin{array}{c}H \quad\ H \\ |\quad\ \ | \\ -C-C- \\ |\quad\ \ | \\ H \quad\ H\end{array}$$

Fig 1.3. Hydrogenation of unsaturated fatty acids

Olive oil is a monounsaturated fatty acid (MUFA). It has been a traditional ingredient of the diet in Mediterranean races for thousands of years. Much has been made of the suggestion that Mediterranean diets should be introduced much more widely to other races to counter coronary heart disease which is low in Mediterraneans. However, other races, such as those of North-West European origin, unfortunately do not have the right genes to benefit from olive oil. It may take a considerable time, anything up to 25 years, before a dietary mistake, similar to that of margarine, is discovered through adverse clinical conditions.

What if Races Intermingle?

Since approximately 1650 the migration of races has escalated throughout the world. How does this affect the genetic diet patterns of the races? As mentioned earlier, it takes roughly a thousand years for a mutation (an error, often spontaneous, in the DNA chemistry) to be accepted and effectively engineered into the intricate data base of man's genetic metabolism (Vogel and Motulsky. *Human Genetics. Problems and Approaches*, 1986). Consequently a man of, for example North-West European origin (British, French, German, Scandinavian, Dutch, Belgian, etc.), the group which has migrated most to distant lands since 1650, should adhere to his basic unrefined North-West European diet to avoid developing metabolic diseases.

If the basic genetic diet of the immigrant does not differ substantially from that of his adopted country, few problems may arise. However, for example, in the case of Africans, with their basic unrefined sorghum diet, emigrating to countries with totally different basic diets, considerable problems will undoubtedly be encountered. This explains the higher incidence of heart disease, hypertension and diabetes among African-Americans in the USA, compared with their white counterparts.

In the case of intermarriage, the descendents of these marriages could inherit either the best or the worst of two dietary legacies.

How Common Are Genetic Mutations?

Genetics is the darling of late 20th-century medicine, and will no doubt swiftly yield a crop of Nobel Prize nominations and winners. High-tech and costly genetic engineering is the subject of much debate and research, while simple issues such as diets and micronutrients are dismissed as food fads for fanatics.

GENETICS: THE HUMAN COMPUTER • 25

Genetic factors consist of chromosomes, 23 pairs in humans, each containing a large number of genes, in total approximately 100 000. These chromosomes and genes contain nucleic acids, nearly all deoxyribonucleic acid (DNA), the latter forming two complementary strands coiled together in a helix. Drs Clark, Wilkens and Watson won the Nobel Prize for

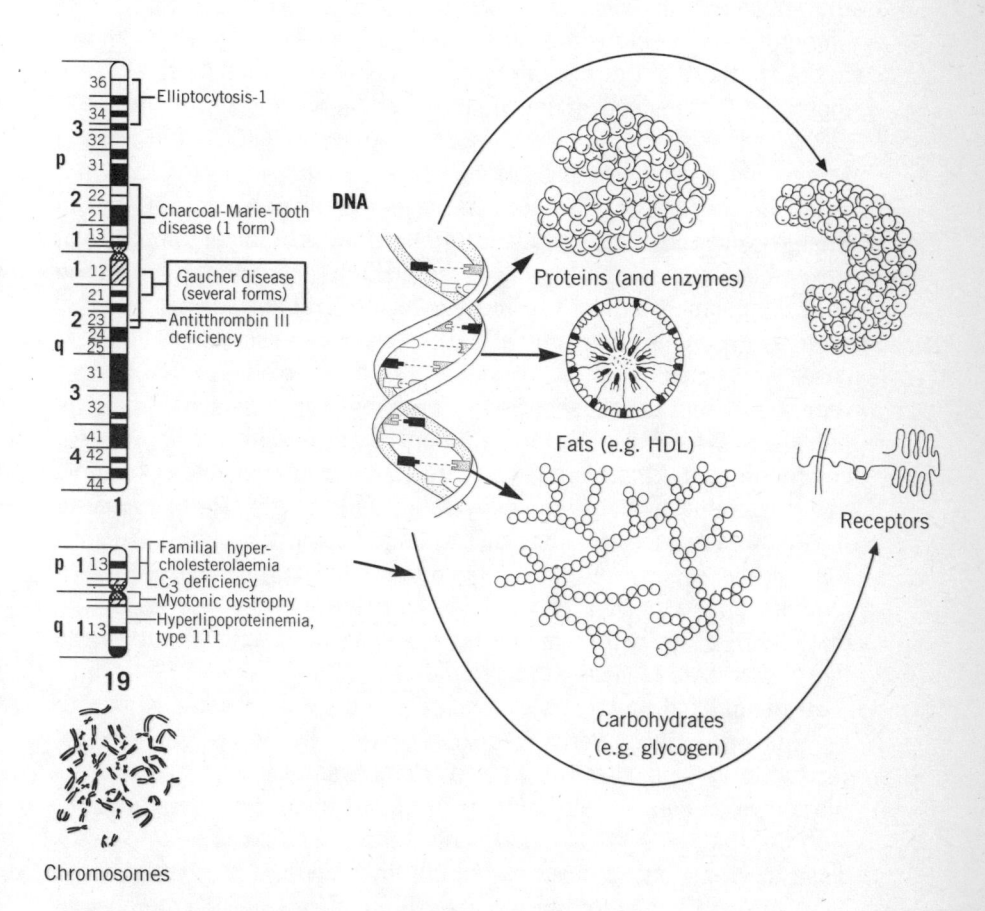

Fig 1.4. An illustration featuring the chromosomes with the positions of some genes on two of the chromosomes (including that of familial hypercholesterolaemia), the helix of DNA, and the formation of proteins, fats, carbohydrates and two forms of receptors.

Medicine in 1962 for discovering this helix structure. It is extremely stable in the face of physical and metabolic agents, yet occasional changes must be able to occur, the so-called mutations. Genes also replicate themselves and their products with extreme precision and accuracy (Fig 1.4). However, some DNAs must differ from one individual to another, as well as from one race or species to another. These facts have frequently been used in legal identification of tissues and blood.

Three main classes of genetic disease are now recognised.
1. Chromosomal disorders. The primary fault lies with the number of chromosomes being either too many or too few. The best-known cases are those of Down's syndrome (mongolism), who have three chromosomes 21, instead of the normal two, appearing in about 1:800 births. Other examples are Turner's syndrome (1:3000 births) and Kleinefelter's syndrome (1:900 births).
2. Mendelian disorders. These cases have typical pedigree patterns in families with sometimes ethnic differences. If the clinical symptoms of the disease are visible but only inherited from one parent, it is known as a dominant disorder. The most common example in this group is *familial hypercholesterolaemia* (FH), a receptor disorder. Patients in cases where heart attacks are frequent in close relatives often believe they suffer from FH, a very serious condition. These persons should be put at ease, for FH is a rare condition, about one in 500 in Western communities. Furthermore FH sufferers always have visible or tangible deposits of cholesterol in the body called xanthomata. These appear in the Achilles tendon, tendons of the hands or on the skin, especially that of the eyelids. A white ring around the cornea of the eye in patients under the age of 40 is frequently present. The far greater majority of cases with a family history of heart attacks is due to the family members following the same diet.

    If the clinical symptoms of a hereditary disease appear only if both parents have the underlying disorder, the inheritance is known as recessive. Wilson's disease, with liver and brain lesions (hepatolenticular degeneration), is one of many examples under this classification.
3. Multifactorial. Here genetic and nongenetic factors combine to cause a disease. All metabolic diseases fall into this group, e.g. atherosclerotic heart disease, hypertension, diabetes mellitus type II, rheumatoid arthritis, etc. It is to this group especially that the comparison to a computer applies, and it is this group that is the main subject of this book.

The metabolic diseases behave as multifactorial conditions when viewed in populations. However, in families it is sometimes possible to identify a single gene fault that is mainly responsible for the disease in that family, e.g. in rheumatoid arthritis.

In Western diseases, alternatively called diseases of civilisation or industrialisation, the partners to genetics in prevention and treatment are micronutrients, i.e. vitamins and minerals. This will be discussed in the next chapter.

How Effective Is an Enzyme Mutation?

Approximately 30% of enzymes can be present in different forms in different persons, races or populations. Two of the most common examples are seen in enzymes controlling milk and alcohol absorption and metabolism (Fig 1.5).

Milk absorption is under control of the enzyme **lactase** in the gut lining. Frequently children and some adults appear unable to absorb milk, and consequently they are labelled "allergic to milk", which is incorrect.

Lactase is found in two almost identical forms, **lactase a** (for the absorption of fresh milk, and found mainly in white races) and **lactase b** (for the absorption of fermented milk, and found almost exclusively in black races).

```
ALCOHOL                                          MILK
   |                                            /    \
Alcohol Dehydrogenase                        Fresh   Fermented
       ADH                                     |        |
      /    \                               Lactase a  Lactase b
   ADH a    ADH b
(effective  (ineffective                  Races       Races
against     against                    originating  originating
alcohol     alcohol                     in colder   in equatorial
toxins)     toxins)                      climates    climates
   |          |
Acetaldehyde Dehydrogenase
         AcDh
      /       \
   AcDH a    AcDH b
(effective  (ineffective
against     against
alcohol     alcohol
toxins)     toxins)

   White
Americans (etc.)   Orientals (etc.)
     85%                85%
```

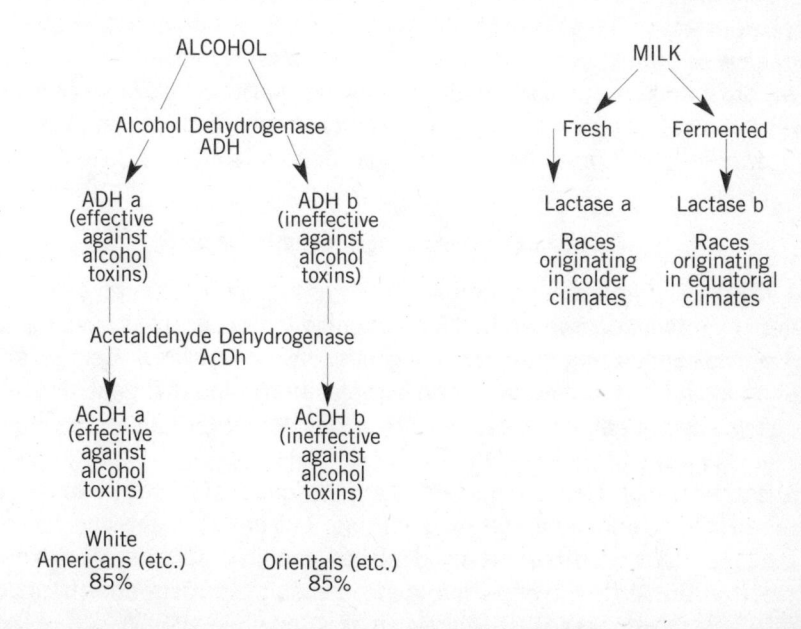

Fig 1.5. The effect of polymorphism of alcohol dehydrogenase, acetaldehyde dehydrogenase and lactase in various races.

The explanation is stunningly simple: lactase b was the original enzyme present in the black races indigenous to the warm equatorial climates. As man gradually migrated to the colder areas nearer the Poles, his skin became lighter, and lactase a developed as a mutation to accommodate fresh milk.

A full examination in populations clearly shows lactase b prominent in equatorial communities, lactase a prominent in colder countries nearer the Poles, while a relatively equal distribution is seen in the in-between areas.

Another wonder of nature is that African babies are able to drink mothers' and fresh cows' milk without any problems. Nature has predetermined through its genetic build-up that, within the first few years of life, a baby belonging to the fermented milk lactase race, will be able to absorb and digest fresh milk. After that nature will rechannel the baby's preference to the form normally used by his race. Nature provides for all emergencies of its own making, but not for those caused by man.

Alcohol tolerance has a similar history to milk tolerance. Two enzymes are affected here, **alcohol dehydrogenase** and **acetaldehyde dehydrogenase**. Here the difference is determined by how long a race has been accustomed or "programmed" to alcohol. The variations in races are similar to those seen in milk intolerance. One example is that 85% of White Americans have those enzymes effective in detoxifying alcohol, while 85% of Orientals have the ineffective enzymes.

We are reminded of some individuals who can drink several bottles or glasses of alcohol with apparent tolerance while others of the same or other races appear to collapse after one or two drinks. It is all in the enzymes.

What Can Be Done about Genetic Diseases?

In the cases of chromosomal and Mendelian disorders, much can be done to relieve symptoms. However, as far as cures are concerned, results are extremely disappointing despite some geneticists' enthusiasm. Genetic engineering, in which the abnormal gene is replaced by a normal gene, is still in the early experimental stages. Results of gene therapy are disappointing (*Science* 1995; 269: 1050-5).

It is known that 100 000 genes determine the growth and development of man. Half the genes have been identified, but unfortunately the function of three-quarters of these genes identified are still completely unknown (*Science* 1995; 270: 368-9). The known genetic disorders are distributed over 767 *loci* in the genes (*J Med Genetics* 1994; 31: 368-9).

However, with regard to multifactorial disorders, the picture is far more favourable. Valuable partners to genetics in this group are the micronutrients, the vitamins and minerals – vital co-factors without which enzymes cannot function adequately.

There is every reason to believe that multifactorial genetic diseases can be cured by replacing the lost micronutrients and applying the correct genetic diet.

CHAPTER 2

MICRONUTRIENTS: SMALL THINGS AND BIG PROBLEMS

The biggest problem in the world could have been solved when it was small.
Walter Bynner

Changing Disease Patterns

Today the average person's ambition is for wealth, health and happiness. Of these three the one that has probably received the most attention but obtained the least results is health. A general and disquieting belief held by many responsible laymen and medical scientists is that man's general health has been deteriorating rather than improving over the last 100 years.

Many factors undoubtedly play a role in this decline in health, and the tendency is to blame overpopulation, malnutrition, smoking, alcoholism, sexual misbehaviour, psychological misdemeanours, etc. Some argue against the view that health has deteriorated. "How can that be? We are living longer than ever before." Granted, statistics indicate that the average lifespan of man has never been longer than at present. However, these statistics include deaths of newborn and other babies, whose figures have decreased considerably in later years. But deaths at the other end of the age scale have not decreased, and in many Western communities have in fact increased. Persons who reached 50 years of age a hundred years ago appeared to live longer on average, compared to those who reached 50 in more recent years (Walker A.R.P., *Postgrad Med J* 1974; 50: 29-32).

When medical journals and textbooks of the later 19th and earlier 20th centuries are scrutinised, it becomes abundantly clear that the disease patterns of those years differ considerably from those of the last 40 to 50 years. What was mainly the era of infective diseases was steadily replaced by atherosclerotic heart disease, high blood pressure, rheumatoid arthritis, diabetes mellitus type II, cancer, osteoporosis, obesity and allergies, amongst others. Some argue that persons of a hundred years ago did not become old enough to develop the above-mentioned newer diseases, but simple statistics disprove that argument.

The question now arises whether these modern diseases could have a common cause. The answer is a most resounding YES.

Two Common Modern Diseases

Two "new" diseases have a similar history, atherosclerotic heart disease and diabetes mellitus type II. In the first mentioned, also known as coronary heart disease (CHD), the only reasonable quantitive measure is the recorded deaths from the disease. In the official *International List of Causes of Deaths*, which is revised periodically, diseases affecting the coronary arteries were classified before 1929 under the general title *Diseases of the Arteries*. Up to that time deaths from heart attacks were so rare that a separate group was not warranted.

In 1929 a new heading was added to the list, *Diseases of the Coronary Arteries and Angina Pectoris*. The incidence was listed as 25.7 per 100 000 population in the USA. In 1938 the listing was changed to *Diseases of the Coronary Arteries*, which has remained unchanged ever since. Those and later listings were as follows:

1929 : 25.7 per 100 000 population.
1938 : 52.2 per 100 000 population.
1940 : 71.3 per 100 000 population.
1945 : 95.8 per 100 000 population.

By 1963 this figure reached the turning point at 307 per 100 000, illustrating a phenomenal twelvefold increase in a short period of 34 years. British figures showed a similar trend. It is appropriate to state here that the year 1963 was when emergency cardiac units came into being, affording better care over the acute stages and saving more lives.

Diabetes appears in two forms: in younger persons the control of the illness is dependent upon insulin injections. In older persons the illness has traditionally been supposed to be the result of overstimulation and exhaustion of the insulin-secreting pancreas, caused in turn by a highly refined carbohydrate diet that includes overindulgence in sugar, confectionery and sweetened beverages. In a comprehensive book, *Two Centuries of American Medicine* by J. Barclay and A.M. Harvey, it is stated that the number of diabetics in the USA increased from 1.2 million in 1950 to an estimated five million in 1975, an increase of more than 300% (or fourfold) over 25 years, while the population increase was only 50%. Between 1980 and 1987 the number again increased – from 5.8 million to 6.8 million. This could not have been due to improved diagnosis as diabetes was never difficult to diagnose.

The Time Factor

Another factor to take into consideration is time. Drs Denis Burkitt and Hugh Trowell, famed pioneers in fibre research and African diseases, declared in their book *Refined Carbohydrate Foods and Diseases*, 1975, that the time required for a disease to become clinically apparent in a race after the introduction of a new environmental factor, is approximately 40 years.

Medically, it requires the acumen of a detective to discover a factor or factors which will support this time claim. Fat, which would be the lipidiologists' favourite, fails the test in Western communities, since the increase in dietary fats took place as far back as the industrial revolution in Britain and elsewhere in the early and middle 19th century. Proteins fail for the same reason.

The one outstanding factor which did coincide accurately with the necessary time factor was the introduction and common use of the roller mills in 1880. Bakers, particularly, searched for a method to whiten their flour. White flour was the food of kings. Previously, to fulfil their aim it is stated that they went to such extreme measures as adding white chalk to their product. No wonder so many constipated decisions were made by the monarchs of old.

Inadvertently, and totally unrealised by anybody at that time, refining had substantially decreased the vital co-factors, vitamins and minerals. Could the loss of these small factors, collectively and appropriately known as micronutrients, have such a major effect on man's health that it could change the whole pattern of disease? Modern medical research strongly supports such a view.

Partners in Perfection

Little doubt exists that minerals have been present since the beginnings of our planet. However, the first appearance of vitamins is far more difficult to determine since, with their more intricate formulas than minerals, their formation was obviously much later (Table 2.1). Nonetheless, from what we know about the functions of vitamins in metabolism, it is obvious that their formation must go back many millions of years.

VITAMINS	MINERALS
Fat Soluble	**Essential above 100 mg per day**
Vitamin A	Calcium
Beta-Carotene	Phosphorous
Vitamin D	Magnesium
Vitamin E	Sodium
Vitamin K	Chloride
	Potassium
Water Soluble	Sulphur
Thiamin (B1)	
Riboflavin (B2)	**Essential at a few mg per day**
Niacin (Nicotinic Acid)	Iron
Vitamin B6 (Pyridoxine)	Zinc
Folic Acid	Copper
Cobalamine (B12)	Iodine
Pantothenic Acid (Coenzyme A)	Manganese
Biotin	Fluoride
Vitamin C	Molybdenum
	Cobalt
Vitamin-like Factors	Selenium
Bioflavonoids	Chromium
Choline	Arsenic
Inositol	Tin
Lipoic Acid	Nickel
Ubiquinone (Coenzyme Q)	Vanadium
	Silicon
Coenzymes	
NAD(P)	
FAD	
ATP (ADP, AMP)	

Table 2.1. Vitamins and minerals in human metabolism.

In the not so distant past of a few hundred years a vitamin shortage condition conjured up a picture of skin lesions, painfully chapped lips, eye opacities, rickets, beri-beri, nerve paralysis, pellagra, etc. These conditions could be considered as the classical signs of vitamin deficiency, which we only see nowadays in excessively severe malnutrition. However, it has lately become clear that a less severe and more chronic vitamin shortage, always accompanied by a similar mineral shortage, could have a far more disastrous effect on man's health than has previously been believed.

This catastrophic development in human health is due to the curbing of normal metabolism, leading to the advent of metabolic diseases. Thanks to the introduction of roller mills in 1880, subsequently helped along by widespread canning and general household refrigeration, man's diet has become grossly depleted of micronutrients, those essential elements of metabolism that have guided the metabolic build-up of man into a direction of normal health for thousands of years.

Metabolic Pathways

Over millions of years, aided by genetics, a well-balanced network of metabolic pathways has developed in man, animal and plant (Table 2.2). Nature, the highly competent but unhurried computer, strives always towards a healthy pattern. It is only from outside interference, such as man believing he can better nature, that problems develop.

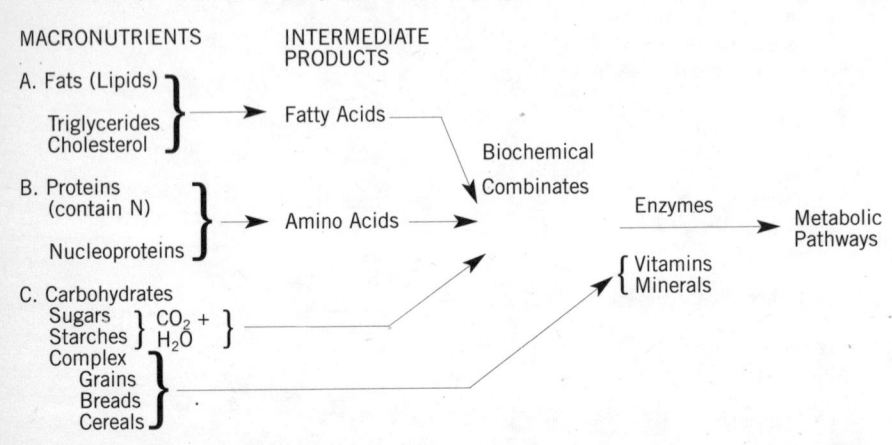

```
MACRONUTRIENTS          INTERMEDIATE
                        PRODUCTS
A. Fats (Lipids)    ⎫
   Triglycerides    ⎬→ Fatty Acids
   Cholesterol      ⎭
                                       Biochemical
B. Proteins         ⎫                  Combines          Enzymes
   (contain N)      ⎬→ Amino Acids  →              →              → Metabolic
   Nucleoproteins   ⎭                        ⎧ Vitamins              Pathways
                                             ⎩ Minerals
C. Carbohydrates
   Sugars    ⎫ CO₂ +
   Starches  ⎭ H₂O
   Complex
     Grains  ⎫
     Breads  ⎬
     Cereals ⎭
```

Table 2.2. Metabolism: A simplified version. Note the important role of complex carbohydrates in providing the greater majority of micronutrients.

The chains of chemical reaction cannot proceed without considerable help. Stimulating every step in the reaction, much larger molecules, the enzymes, which are all proteins, were required. Now the reaction speeded up considerably but nature was not yet satisfied with the pace. A further stimulant was necessary. Now the most important function of micronutrients was to be realised. They became the co-factors of enzymes, essential in speeding up the whole metabolic pathway to an incredible rate of approximately 4 000 molecules forming per second. Vitamins and minerals virtually became partners in perfection. This reaction is illustrated in Fig 2.1.

Biochemists have met regularly through the years to discus new enzymes, their functions and their co-factors. In 1961 only 721 enzymes had been discovered, but by 1984 a total of 2 477 enzymes were recorded, and it was believed that few if any more existed. Of these enzymes approximately 60% also had their co-factors or micronutrients established (Webb E.C., *International Congress on Enzymes*, IUB, 1984).

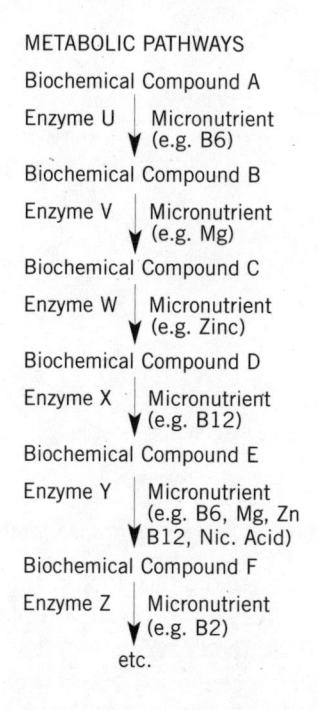

```
           METABOLIC PATHWAYS
           Biochemical Compound A
           Enzyme U  | Micronutrient
                     ▼ (e.g. B6)
           Biochemical Compound B
           Enzyme V  | Micronutrient
                     ▼ (e.g. Mg)
           Biochemical Compound C
           Enzyme W  | Micronutrient
                     ▼ (e.g. Zinc)
           Biochemical Compound D
           Enzyme X  | Micronutrient
                     ▼ (e.g. B12)
           Biochemical Compound E
           Enzyme Y  | Micronutrient
                     | (e.g. B6, Mg, Zn
                     ▼  B12, Nic. Acid)
           Biochemical Compound F
           Enzyme Z  | Micronutrient
                     ▼ (e.g. B2)
                 etc.
```

Fig 2.1. Demonstrating metabolic pathways and the action of enzymes and micronutrients.

To identify which micronutrients are needed for each specific enzyme is a tedious and difficult procedure, each enzyme frequently requiring a large number of experiments to determine which of the approximately 40 micronutrients speed up the reaction. Consequently this line of research has been largely curtailed, all biochemists being satisfied that all enzymes require micronutrients. Those not yet discovered will eventually be found.

At present we can use a round figure of 2 500 as the number of known enzymes.

Two disease patterns are therefore seen with a shortage of vitamins and minerals (Fig 2.2).

1. Acute shortages, usually associated with malnutrition, leading to the classic conditions of beri-beri, pellagra, etc.
2. Chronic shortages over much longer periods of perhaps up to 40 or 50 years or longer since birth, leading to metabolic diseases. This group now undoubtedly presents the greater number of modern diseases seen in medical practice.

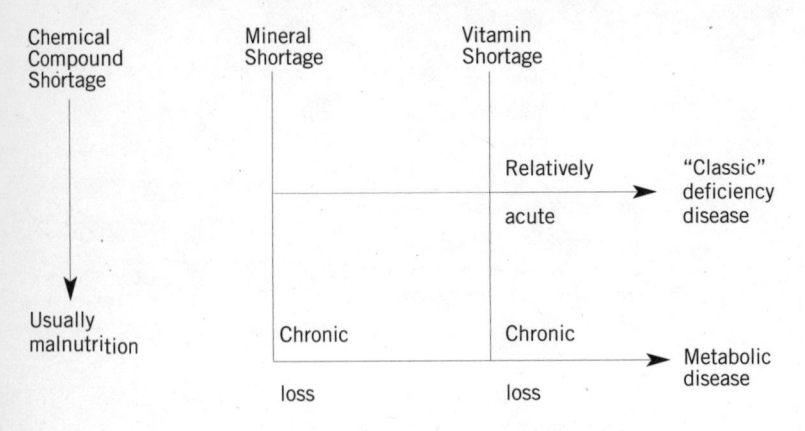

```
Chemical            Mineral              Vitamin
Compound            Shortage             Shortage
Shortage
                                         Relatively        "Classic"
                                                           deficiency
                                         acute             disease

   ▼
Usually             Chronic              Chronic
malnutrition                                               Metabolic
                                                           disease
                    loss                 loss
```

Fig 2.2. Result of micronutrient loss. Note the difference in results due to a relatively acute loss and a chronic loss.

The Extent of Dietary Micronutrient Loss

Although the concentration of micronutrients in foods before the advent of roller mills in 1880 is unknown, a reasonably good estimation can be obtained if the most unrefined foods available today can be compared to the most refined. This loss is especially notable in grain foods such as wheat, bread, rice and maize (corn). The actual differences are probably slightly higher, as the most unrefined grains commercially available have already undergone a degree of refinement (Table 2.3).

Simple arithmetic informs us that in the refining process of the above grains, up to 50% micronutrients are lost in 82% of grains, up to 60% are lost in 68% of grains, up to 70% are lost in 47% of grains, up to 80% are lost in 28% of grains, and between 81% and 100% are lost in 19% of grains.

Little doubt can therefore be expressed about the fact that the body's metabolism must be seriously affected, and that the effect eventually leads to metabolic diseases.

	Loss in white bread (a)	Loss in white rice (b)	Loss in super maize (c)	RDA males 25-50 yrs
Fibre	-69%	-48%	-75%	
Calcium	-20%	-16%	-70%	800 mg
Iron	-60%	-60%	-83%	10 mg
Magnesium	-68%	-93%	-74%	350 mg
Phosphate	-45%	-62%	-66%	800 mg
Potassium	-47%	-62%	-56%	?
Zinc	-55%	-40%	-78%	15 mg
Copper	-62%	-75%	-70%	1.5-3 mg
Manganese	-76%	-70%	-86%	2.0-5 mg
Thiamine (B1)	-31%	-78%	-60%	1.5 mg
Riboflavine (B2)	-42%	-50%	-70%	1.7 mg
Niacin (Nic. Acid)	-60%	-71%	-73%	19 mg
Pyridoxin (B6)	-73%	-80%	-87%	2 mg
Folic Acid	-32%	0	-58%	0.2 mg
Biotin	-84%	-75%	-54%	30-100 ug
Vitamin A	0*	0*	0*	1000 ug RE
Vitamin D	0*	0*	0*	5 ug
Vitamin E	0*	-54%	-62%	10 mg
Vitamin C	0*	0*	0*	60 mg

(a) Loss compared to white bread
(b) Loss compared to brown rice
(c) Loss compared to straight-run raw maize
* Indicates 100% loss in unrefined form commercially available
RDA: Recommended dietary allowance per day
Table 2.3. Percentage losses of micronutrients in food refining
(References: *Compositions of Foods, Agricultural Handbook No 8*, 1975 and 1984, USA; *MRC Food Composition Tables*, 3rd edition, Langenhoven et al., Parow, 1991).

The Refining of Sorghum

It has already been noted that sorghum was the basic food of the African for approximately 3 500 years. In Africa sorghum has largely lost the commercial battle against maize, the latter nearly exclusively in the refined form. In America, the African, mainly descended from imported slaves, has largely adopted a Western diet similar to that of the North-West European or Mediterranean descendents in America.

It is important to compare the concentrations of micronutrients in sorghum, refined maize and unrefined maize (Table 2.4). The well-established difference in low incidence of osteoporosis in people of African origin compared to the high incidence in people of North-West European origin could have its cause in the differences of calcium, magnesium and phosphorous in these grains.

	White super raw maize	Straight-run raw maize	Maltabella uncooked
	per 100 g		
Total fat (g)	1.2	4.3	2.5
Total carbohydrate (g)	83.5	75.1	72.0
Fibre (g)	2.6	10.6	1.5
Calcium (mg)	3.0	10.0	21.0
Magnesium (mg)	32.0	123.0	117.0
Phosphate (mg)	71.0	241.0	192.0
Zinc (mg)	0.5	2.3	2.64
Thiamine (mg)	0.2	0.5	0.46
Riboflavine (mg)	0.03	0.12	0.15
Nicotinic Acid (mg)	0.6	2.2	3.9

Table 2.4. A comparison of some of the contents of refined maize, unrefined maize and Maltabella (sorghum). Note particularly the gross loss of calcium, magnesium and zinc. (Reference: *MRC Food Composition Tables*, 3rd edition, Langenhoven et al., Parow, 1991.)

The unrefined forms of maize and sorghum are commercially extremely rare due to the misguided common preference for the refined forms. However, they can be obtained by directly approaching the mills concerned. Refrigeration is necessary to preserve these grains.

CHAPTER 3

THE AMAZING WORLD OF FATTY ACIDS

It cannot be too often repeated that it is not help but obstacles, not facilities but difficulties, that make man.

W. MATTHEWS, AMERICAN AUTHOR (1818-1909)

Introduction

If you are one who dislikes difficult explanations, even if it is essential in the battle against major causes of ill-health, then skip this chapter. However, if you wish to gain insight and knowledge into the intricacies of man's most delicate computer in maintaining good health, then join us in reading further.

The field of fatty acids is one of the most controversial in modern medicine. The layman's knowledge stretches little beyond a propaganda-instilled view of saturated and unsaturated fatty acids, with the impression that saturates are wholly animal fats which are harmful to his health, and that the unsaturates are wholly vegetable fats which will save him from heart attacks. These views, vigorously supported by unscrupulous commercial interests are, in their entirety, incorrect. Table 3.1. illustrates that animal and vegetable fats are only proportionately saturated and unsaturated. Eating polyunsaturated fatty acids is nothing new; man has been eating them for thousands of years.

But first, what is a fatty acid? All fats, alternatively called lipids, either contain or are related to fatty acids. Fatty acids appear as chains in space

	Total fat	Sat. fat	%	MU fat	%	PU fat	%	Chol
	g/100 g							mg/100 g
Beef, fried rump steak (fat trimmed)	7.4	3.04	41	3.44	46	0.29	4	82
Fatty fish, medium fat, steamed	3.7	0.99	27	1.17	32	1.35	36	80
Margarine, hard	81.0	18.55	23	41.44	51	17.10	21	0
Margarine, soft	81.0	16.00	20	26.95	33	34.06	42	0
Butter	81.0	45.09	56	20.36	25	1.60	2	219

Sat. = Saturated; MU = Monounsaturated; PU = Polyunsaturated

Table 3.1. A comparison in fat content of five commonly used foods. Note that there is no clear-cut differentiation in fatty acids between animal fats and vegetable fats.

containing anything from two to 24 carbon (C) atoms, the latter in multiples of two. The important fatty acids in man contain 16 carbon atoms or more. A saturated bond between two carbon atoms is indicated by a single line or dash, and an unsaturated bond by a double line or dash. A shorthand designation has been devised for indicating composition in terms of the number of carbon atoms and double bonds, as well as the position of unsaturated bonds from the carboxyl (COOH) end (Table 3.2). The three-dimensional form of the fatty acids in space is important from the viewpoint of genetics.

COMPONENTS	TRIVIAL NAME
2:0	Acetic acid
16:0	Palmitic acid
18:0	Stearic acid
18:1 (9)	Oleic acid
18:1 (11)	Vaccenic acid
18:2 (9,12)	Linoleic acid
18:3 (9,12,15)	Linolenic (alpha) acid
20:4 (5.8,11,14)	Arachidonic acid

Table 3.2. Some fatty acids and their shorthand designations.

The most common saturated fatty acid is palmitic acid.

H_3C_{16} ⋯⋯ $_1$ COOH   16:0

The most common unsaturated fatty acid is linoleic acid.

H_3C_{18} ⋯⋯ ^{1} COOH   18:2 (9,12)

Essential Fatty Acid Metabolism

Two of the most common fatty acids in the body are cislinoleic acid, 18:2 (9, 12) and alpha-linolenic acid, 18:3 (9, 12, 15). But more important, they are also known as essential fatty acids. What is essential about them? The problem is resolved if it is realised that they are essential dietary fatty acids, i.e. their only origin is in the diet, and they cannot be sufficiently formed in the body for use.

To complicate matters, two linoleic acids exist, the other being gamma-linoleinic acid (GLA; some may recollect the name Efamol, for that is what it is).

THE AMAZING WORLD OF FATTY ACIDS • 41

To complicate matters still further, an alternate nomenclature has developed, that of omega, the latter being-Greek for *end*. In this case the methyl (CH_2) end is indicated. Omega-3 indicates that the first unsaturated bond is at the third carbon atom from the CH end and the omega-6 indicates the sixth unsaturated bond from the CH_2 end. The latter omega nomenclature also has a shorthand designation.

The importance of differentiating between these two similar fatty acids is that they represent two totally different genetic pathways developed from different species of animal, including man.

In no other field of dietary genetics is the biochemistry so sensitively balanced as in that of essential fatty acids and their derivatives: prostaglandins, leukotrienes and thromboxanes (Fig 3.1). Not only do they represent separate

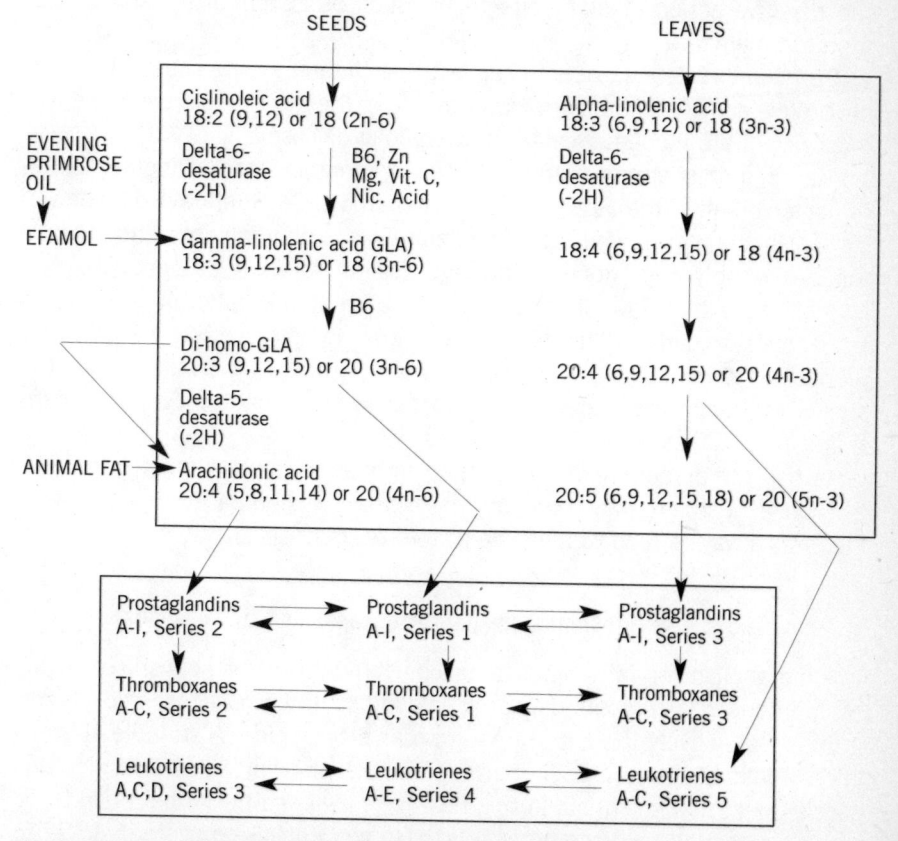

```
                            SEEDS                         LEAVES
                              ↓                             ↓
              ┌─────────────────────────────────────────────────────────────┐
              │  Cislinoleic acid              Alpha-linolenic acid         │
              │  18:2 (9,12) or 18 (2n-6)      18:3 (6,9,12) or 18 (3n-3)   │
 EVENING      │  Delta-6-        B6, Zn        Delta-6-                     │
 PRIMROSE     │  desaturase      Mg, Vit. C,   desaturase                   │
 OIL          │  (-2H)           Nic. Acid     (-2H)                        │
   ↓          │     ↓                             ↓                         │
 EFAMOL ────→ │  Gamma-linolenic acid GLA)     18:4 (6,9,12,15) or 18 (4n-3)│
              │  18:3 (9,12,15) or 18 (3n-6)                                │
              │        ↓ B6                                                 │
              │  Di-homo-GLA                                                │
              │  20:3 (9,12,15) or 20 (3n-6)   20:4 (6,9,12,15) or 20 (4n-3)│
              │  Delta-5-                                                   │
              │  desaturase                                                 │
              │  (-2H)                                                      │
 ANIMAL FAT→  │  Arachidonic acid                                           │
              │  20:4 (5,8,11,14) or 20 (4n-6) 20:5 (6,9,12,15,18) or 20 (5n-3)│
              └─────────────────────────────────────────────────────────────┘
                    ↓              ↓                    ↓
              ┌─────────────────────────────────────────────────────────────┐
              │  Prostaglandins  → Prostaglandins  →  Prostaglandins        │
              │  A-I, Series 2  ←  A-I, Series 1   ←  A-I, Series 3         │
              │       ↓                 ↓                  ↓                │
              │  Thromboxanes   → Thromboxanes     →  Thromboxanes          │
              │  A-C, Series 2  ← A-C, Series 1    ←  A-C, Series 3         │
              │       ↓                 ↓                  ↓                │
              │  Leukotrienes   → Leukotrienes     →  Leukotrienes          │
              │  A,C,D, Series 3 ← A-E, Series 4   ←  A-C, Series 5         │
              └─────────────────────────────────────────────────────────────┘
```

Fig 3.1. The metabolism of essential fatty acids, prostaglandins, thromboxanes and leukotrienes. This should be seen as genetic programming in delicately balanced metabolism.

pathways necessary for leaves, seeds and animal origins, but the loss of micronutrients considerably aggravates matters further. The cat family lived nearly exclusively from meat, the antelope family exclusively from leaves and grass, while man followed a mixed animal and seed diet. Nature's computer, via fatty acids, has allowed for this, but any drastic or chronic change will not lead to a hurried adaptation – indeed, it would take a thousand years.

Central to the micronutrients' role in this metabolism is the enzyme **delta-6-desaturase** which requires five micronutrients for its normal action, vitamin B6, vitamin C, magnesium, zinc, and nicotinic acid (niacin) (*Med Hypothesis* 1980; 6: 785-800, *Med Hypothesis* 1994; 42: 149-58). This enzyme regulates the reaction cislinoleic acid to gamma-linolenic acid, as well as alpha-linolenic acid to the next step in the omega-3 pathway. It is very sensitive to the negative action of many chemicals, such as abnormal transfatty acids found in margarine.

Sufficient evidence exists to suggest that the imbalance caused by a loss of the five above-mentioned micronutrients is the key to the development of most, if not all, modern Western or metabolic diseases.

Man requires approximately six times more of the cislinoleic family (omega-6) than of the alpha-linolenic one (omega-3). Sunflower oil contains 54% cislinoleic acid, while grass contains 64% alpha-linolenic acid. The cat family probably does not have delta-6-desaturase as it does not need it. Human races that have traditionally not eaten animal fats but live on fish alone, such as certain Canadian Indians, also do not have this enzyme. It is probable that the Eskimos have no delta-5-desaturase, otherwise needed two stages further in the metabolism (Sinclair H.M., *Omega-6 Essential Fatty Acids*, p. 1-20, 1990).

In fish the predominant unsaturated fatty acids contain mainly omega-3 20 and 22 carbons, factors which have proved beneficial to man's health. Fish was always a food of man, be it from rivers or seas.

The "Eics" (Prostaglandins, Thromboxanes and Leukotrienes)

The metabolism of fatty acids proceeds through to the network of highly "computerised" compounds, prostaglandins, thromboxanes and leukotrienes. Collectively the latter are known as eicosanoids. A suitable abbreviation would be "eics". So important did the medical world consider this development that scientists in this field were awarded the Nobel Prize twice within a period of ten years; in 1973 to Ulf von Euler, and again in 1982 to Sune Bergström, Bengst Samuelson and John Vane.

Eics are formed in three series of fatty acids. Each series develops in separate pathways from three fatty acids, cislinoleic acid (series 1), arachidonic acid (series 2) and alpha-linolenic acid (series 3). Each series of prostaglandins has nine subgroups A to I. Each thromboxane series has 3 subgroups A to C. Leukotrienes have three series C, D and E, with odd subgroups amongst them. Some of these subgroups are further divided. We therefore have a minimum total of $(9 \times 3) + (3 \times 3) + (3 + 5 + 3)$, at least 47 eics.

Function of Eics

In a nutshell, eics control virtually every physiological function in the body. They consist of small hormone-like molecules of molecular weights approximately 350 (albumin, a relatively small protein has a molecular weight of 69 000), and restrict their functions to within the cells or in the latter's immediate surroundings. Eics function in opposite pairs or multiples thereof, with the effect of attempting to balance each other out. They vary in different animals, thereby complicating animal experiments designed for application to humans.

Resembling science fiction, there are literaly hundreds of thousands of eics in nearly every cell in the body. Instead of listing the numerous functions and interactions of the eics, which would fill many pages of this book, Fig 3.2 illustrates a very small fraction of the functions of eics in different organs or tissues of the body. A sense of intercomputer connections is to be imagined. There is no doubt that further interaction with genetics exists.

Consequences of Eics Imbalances

With the knowledge that eics control virtually all physiological functions of the body, the following reasonable conclusions can be made:
1. The loss of micronutrients necessary for the normal function of delta-6-desaturase must inevitably lead to a shortage of the series 1 eics, including certain leukotrienes, and therefore to an imbalance of eics.
2. Any short-term imbalance of eics will lead to abnormal physiological functions. It would be difficult to define these changes because they may be of short duration. Certain allergies, such as asthma, hay fever and urticaria (a skin condition), may be examples.
3. Of far greater importance is that these imbalances and shortages are

44 • A BLUEPRINT FOR BETTER HEALTH

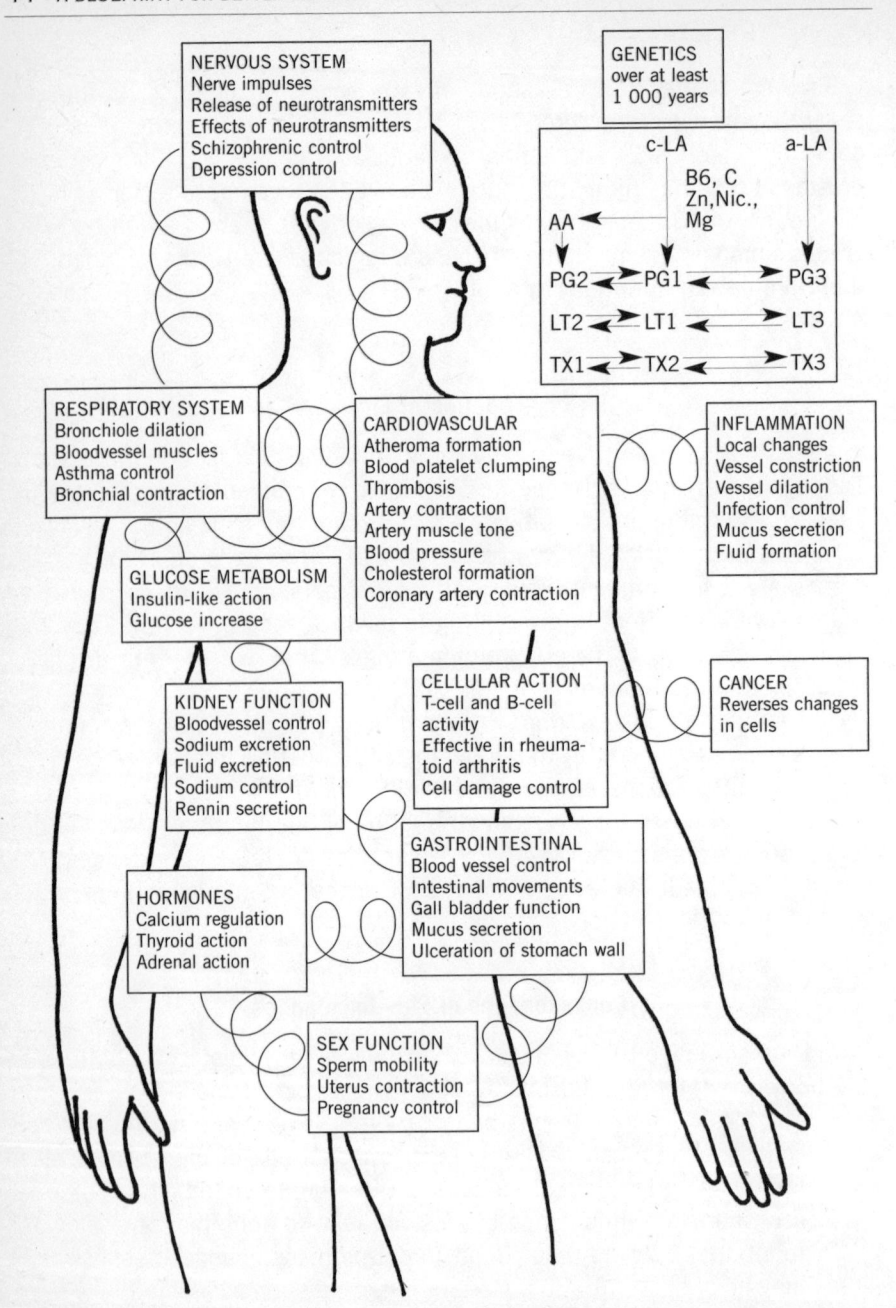

NERVOUS SYSTEM
Nerve impulses
Release of neurotransmitters
Effects of neurotransmitters
Schizophrenic control
Depression control

GENETICS
over at least
1 000 years

c-LA　　　　　　a-LA
　　　B6, C
　　　Zn, Nic.,
　　　Mg
AA
↓
PG2 ⇌ PG1 ⇌ PG3
LT2 ⇌ LT1 ⇌ LT3
TX1 ⇌ TX2 ⇌ TX3

RESPIRATORY SYSTEM
Bronchiole dilation
Bloodvessel muscles
Asthma control
Bronchial contraction

CARDIOVASCULAR
Atheroma formation
Blood platelet clumping
Thrombosis
Artery contraction
Artery muscle tone
Blood pressure
Cholesterol formation
Coronary artery contraction

INFLAMMATION
Local changes
Vessel constriction
Vessel dilation
Infection control
Mucus secretion
Fluid formation

GLUCOSE METABOLISM
Insulin-like action
Glucose increase

KIDNEY FUNCTION
Bloodvessel control
Sodium excretion
Fluid excretion
Sodium control
Rennin secretion

CELLULAR ACTION
T-cell and B-cell activity
Effective in rheuma-toid arthritis
Cell damage control

CANCER
Reverses changes in cells

GASTROINTESTINAL
Blood vessel control
Intestinal movements
Gall bladder function
Mucus secretion
Ulceration of stomach wall

HORMONES
Calcium regulation
Thyroid action
Adrenal action

SEX FUNCTION
Sperm mobility
Uterus contraction
Pregnancy control

Fig 3.2. A small fraction of the functions of the eics. Note that the functions are interlinked with each other, the micronutrients and genetics, suggesting the action of a human computer.

usually of a longer period, perhaps a lifetime. This points strongly to an extremely important factor in the development of all metabolic diseases, by far the most common diseases of present civilisation.
4. Imbalances can also develop as a result of foodstuffs which cannot follow the normal genetic pathways of specific genetic races. These can be basic foodstuffs fed to the wrong genetic race, or commercial foodstuffs that are either new or have undergone such alterations that they cannot be metabolised along the normal genetic pathways.
5. Delta-6-desaturase, an important rate-regulating enzyme, necessitating the co-factor function of at least five micronutrients, can itself be absent if, as a result of genetics, this pathway is neither necessary nor utilised, as in the cat family for example.
6. A number of factors, such as transfatty acids (as in margarine), ageing, diabetes and alcohol, may inhibit delta-6-desaturase function.

The Metabolic Diseases

By definition, these are a group of diseases developing as a result of disturbances in the metabolic pathways. The fault can either be in an enzyme or, more likely, due to a loss of micronutrients. Genetics play a vital role in primary enzyme diseases which though plentiful with 928 disorders described (*J Med Genetics* 1994; 31: 265-79), are all rare as individual diseases. Specialised textbooks should be consulted.

Micronutrient shortage diseases must be considered as the most common diseases of present-day medicine, and every indication is that they are on the increase. These diseases are also referred to as "Western" diseases. This is a nondefinitive nomenclature for "how far west must you go?"

Alternatively the terms "civilised" or "industrialised" could be utilised. But civilised is a relative term and could be related to times indefinitely. Industrialisation took place 150 to 200 years ago, long before these diseases made their entries. To finalise, metabolic diseases would be the definitively correct term.

Four famous researchers have listed what they consider metabolic (Western, civilised, industrial) diseases, Prof M.H. Sinclair (1990, *Omega-6 Essential Fatty Acids*), Surgeon-Captain T.L. Cleave (1974, *The Saccharine Disease*), and Drs Denis Burkitt and Hugh Trowell (1975, *Refined Carbohydrate Foods and Disease*). Table 3.3 summarises these lists.

	S	B&T	C
Artherosclerosis + CHD	X	X	X
Pulmonary embolism	X		X
Cerebrovascular disease	X		
Hypertension			X
Lung cancer	X		
Stomach cancer	X		
Peptic ulcer	X		X
Appendicitis	X		X
Ulcerative colitis	X	X	
Gall stones	X	X	
Crohn's disease	X	X	
Diverticulitis	X	X	X
Cholycystitis	X	X	X
Haemorrhoids		X	X
Hiatus hernia		X	X
Cancer of colon			X
Constipation			X
Diabetes mellitus type II	X	X	X
Varicose veins		X	X
Deep venous thrombosis		X	
Multiple sclerosis	X	X	
Rheumatoid arthritis	X	X	
Still's disease		X	
Ankylosing spondylitis		X	
Slipped discs	X		
Collagen (mesenchymal) diseases	X	X	
Systemic lupus erythernatosis	X	X	
Sjogrens disease		X	
Scleroderma		X	
Osteoporosis	X		
Leukaemia	X		
Dental caries	X		X
Nephrosis	X		
Renal stones	X		
Pre-eclampsia	X		
Acne vulgaris	X		
Acne rosacea			X
Asthma	X		
Hypercalcaemia in infants	X		
Certain virus infections (+ polio)	X		
Varicocoele			X
Periodontitis			X
Obesity			X
Primary cystitis			X

Table 3.3. A list of metabolic ("Western") diseases as listed by H.M. Sinclair, 1990 (S), Burkitt and Trowell, 1975 (B&T) and T.L. Cleave, 1974 (C).

The author does not necessarily agree with the inclusion of all the above as metabolic diseases, but by far the larger percentage do fall under this category. A few additional conditions, however, could be included, such as hay fever, allergic skin conditions and myelofibrosis of the bone marrow.

Some Important Recessive Genetic Factors

A number of genetic factors which have an extra impact on metabolic diseases have been known for some time, while others have only become known lately.

Human lymphocytic antigens (HLA) is the most important histocompatibility complex in the body, i.e. they indicate the chances of transplanted material, such as heart, kidneys and skin, to be retained successfully by the body or not. Furthermore, susceptibility to over 40 diseases has been linked to different HLA types in man. This is clearly seen in certain diseases of an auto-immune nature affecting a range of organ systems, including joints (rheumatoid arthritis), the gut, the liver, the kidneys, the glands (including insulin-dependent diabetes mellitus) and the nervous system (including multiple sclerosis) (Bell J.I., *Advances in Human Genetics 18*, 1989).

Genetic lipoproteins (fats combined with proteins) are present. The protein part, known as apoproteins, have different types, three Apo-As, one Apo-B, three Apo-Cs, one Apo-D and three Apo-Es. Lipoprotein small a, or (a), is genetically inherited and found to be increased in genetic races that have a high susceptibility to heart attacks (Zannis V.I., *Advances in Human Genetics 14*, 1985; Editorial *Lancet*, Feb. 16, 1991).

Stress or heart-shock proteins and fibroblast growth factors are further recent discoveries. The first is protective against high temperatures and other stressful stimulants, and probably play an important role in protection against auto-immune diseases, especially rheumatoid arthritis and systemic lupus erythematosis (Editorial *Lancet*, Feb. 19, 1991). At least seven fibroblast growth factors are known, which may effect atherosclerosis, diabetes, cancers (breast, bladder, liver, brain), brain and nerves, eyes, kidneys and heart muscle. It is likely that they play a role in the development of Alzheimer's, Parkinson's and Huntingdon's diseases (*Lancet*, Sept. 29, 1990).

Yet despite all these recessive genetic factors, it is reasonable to believe that in the presence of optimum micronutrients, either per diet and/or per supplementation, the effects of these genetic factors could be so suppressed that their effects are negligible or only of minor importance.

Fatty Acids Let Loose Are Fatal

It must be obvious to the reader by now that all chemical substances, including fats and fatty acids, metabolise according to strict rules and rigid pathways. As the "epidemic" of heart attacks increased in the Fifties, medical scientists took, albeit with good intentions, some questionable action to quell this dreaded disease. It must also be remembered that all the causative facts about heart disease had not yet been discovered, and scientists had to act on what they believed was correct. As ever, the public demanded it.

It must also be stressed, though, that commercial companies took a notoriously self-interested stand, and that financial profits were frequently uppermost in their minds. Commerce had the means of influencing scientists to support theories that advanced their financial gains.

Commercial interests were first mooted when the Seven Countries Study researchers announced that, in order that to reverse the alarming rise in deaths from heart attacks, a swop from animal to vegetable fats and fatty acids, especially polyunsaturates, should be made. The margarine industry rose to the occasion and flooded the medical profession with propaganda. Later, when it was realised that blood cholesterols had to be lowered, the pharmaceutical industry inundated the market with drugs that either decreased the absorption of cholesterol in the gut, or directly interfered with the body's formation of the absolutely essential cholesterol.

In an upsurge of "something has to be done", a new critical value of 5.2 mmol/l for total blood cholesterol, based purely on arbitrary decisions with no proof whatsoever, was hailed as the value separating the heart attack risk cases from the "desirable" values. The decision to choose this value was based on the fact that 40% of the American population fell below this value, but why only 40% should be considered normal and 60% abnormal and at risk is anybody's guess. It not only boosted vegetable oil, margarine and pharmaceutical sales but also invigorated certain relevant medical interests, such as dieticians, pathologists, cardiologists and heart surgeons. All possible means were to be applied to lower the blood cholesterol values to below the magic life-saving figure of 5.2 mmol/l or 200 mg%. The latter is a nice round figure.

Circumstances Leading to the Lipid Theory

A method for cholesterol estimation was first described in 1885. Since then the methodology has so improved that individual laboratories can estimate hundreds of cholesterol values every day. In 1908 a Russian A.I. Ignatowski was the first to suggest that atherosclerosis was of dietary origin. While performing postmortems on his patients, as was frequently the custom of medical practitioners then, he discovered that his rich patients all had atherosclerosis, but very little was noted in his poorer patients. In experiments on rabbits he discovered that a high protein diet led to atherosclerosis. Consequently he claimed that proteins were the cause of atherosclerosis.

In 1913 two more Russians, N. Anitschkow and S. Chalatow, fed rabbits a high cholesterol diet, thus also causing atherosclerosis. So the lipid theory was born. Later it will be shown that, on re-examination of the two sets of slides made in the two above experiments, marked differences were noted. The protein slides resembled very much the later development of atherosclerosis, while the lipid slides showed an infiltration of lipids outside the blood vessels more resembling the picture of familial hypercholesterolaemia, which is a genetic disease of cholesterol.

However the lipid researchers won the day and received the most support. If cholesterol is increased inside the blood vessels it must come from the cholesterol in the diet. How otherwise would cholesterol get there? Dr Ancel Keys, a prominent physiologist and later epidemiologist from the USA, initiated the Seven Countries Study (USA, Japan, Greece, Italy, Netherlands, Yugoslavia, Finland) in 1955 with the primary motive of defining the causes of the increasing heart-death rate.

But alas, Keys had decided from the start that fats/lipids were the offenders, so he limited his study to the dietary lipids, especially the fatty acids (Table 3.4).

Country	Saturated fatty acids	Monounsat. fatty acids	Polyunsat. fatty acids	Total
Kyushuo, Japan	3	3	3	9
Velika Krsna, Serbia	9	12	3	24
Montegiorgio, Italy	9	13	3	25
Crevalcore, Italy	10	14	3	27
Dalmatia	9	16	7	32
Slavonija	14	16	3	33
Corfu	7	22	4	33
West Finland	19	13	3	35
East Finland	22	14	3	39
Crete	8	29	3	40
Zutphen, Netherlands	19	16	5	40
US Railroad	17-18	17-18	4-6	40

Table 3.4. Average percentage of kilojoules from fats, men 40-59 years, from the Seven Countries Study.

His conclusions were that saturated fatty acids were high in the diets of countries with a high incidence of heart deaths, while polyunsaturated fats were high in the diets of countries with a low heart-death rate. Thus the conclusion that polyunsaturated vegetable fats are a good thing and saturated animal fats are a bad thing.

Keys's blatant mistakes were of a threefold order:
1. He never looked at fibre (which he admits in a later book), proteins, amino acids, carbohydrates, vitamins and minerals, but concentrated only on fats. The majority of potential risk factors were thus omitted.
2. Limiting his study initially to a small number of years, he failed to note the general trend per capita intake of the individual fatty acid groups in the years prior to and since the initiation of the study. This indicated a decrease of saturated animal fats in the USA per capita and an increase of unsaturated vegetable fats in the USA per capita while deaths from heart attacks were increasing. (See later for more detail.)
3. Genetic factors were not taken into consideration. The USA, Netherlands and Finland were mainly from the North-West European race; Greece, Italy and Yugoslavia from the Mediterranean race and Japan from the Sino-Japanese. The fats and fatty acids differed genetically in these three groups.

Dietary Recommendations of the American Heart Association (AHA)

Based on the very incomplete Seven Countries Study, the AHA published recommendations for lowering heart attack incidences over a number of years. Between 1961 and 1968 they recommended, besides weight regulation and regular moderate exercise, that the total dietary fat be restricted to 30-35% of total energy, with an equal percentage (10%) of saturated, monounsaturated and polyunsaturated fats. This decision on equal distribution of fats is extremely difficult to comprehend from the Seven Countries Study. Was it because the Japanese, with their low incidence, had an equal distribution of 3% of the three types of fat, that it was concluded that an equal distribution of 10% would be as beneficial? The difference between 3% and 10% is more than threefold. The genetic dietary factors were obviously not considered.

A further AHA recommendation was that the total cholesterol intake should not exceed 300 mg per day. Certainly most of the countries with low coronary heart deaths had low cholesterol intakes, while the USA had an average intake nearer 450 mg per day. But what about the role of genetics?

Races habituated to a high cholesterol intake for 30 to 40 generations have the genetic mechanism to control their cholesterol metabolism to minimise heart attacks. Obviously races with a low cholesterol intake for generations (such as Japanese and Africans, amongst others) have little control over their cholesterol metabolism and develop heart attacks at lower blood cholesterol levels than in North-West European descendents.

In 1973 the AHA made its first commonsense recommendation, albeit unwittingly, that dietary complex carbohydrates (mainly fibres and grains) should be increased to 55% of the total energy intake. Although primarily implying an increase in fibre, it inadvertently led to an increase of dietary micronutrients, the main factor in controlling the level of blood cholesterol. How is this possible? Cholesterol consists of one-third free cholesterol and two-thirds cholesterol-esters. Esters are chemical combinations with fatty acids. The main fatty acid in cholesterol-esters is cislinoleic acid, 55% of the total, the same essential fatty acid previously reported as requiring five micronutrients necessary for its breakdown. Furthermore at least 11 other fatty acids, eight of which are subject to micronutrient control, are also present in cholesterol-esters. Later it will be shown in more detail how micronutrients are the most important factors in controlling blood cholesterol levels (Fig 3.3).

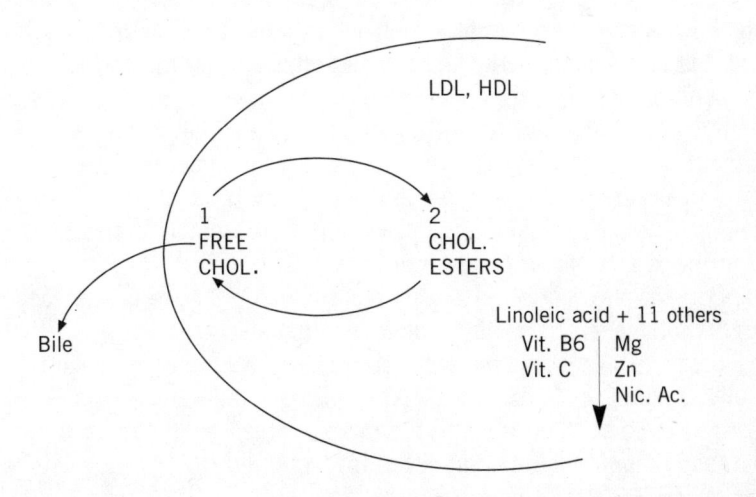

LDL, HDL

1
FREE
CHOL.

2
CHOL.
ESTERS

Linoleic acid + 11 others
Vit. B6	Mg
Vit. C	Zn
	Nic. Ac.

Bile

Fig 3.3. Micronutrient control of blood cholesterol. This occurs in both LDL and HDL. Linoleic acid content is 50-55% of total cholesterol esters. Only free cholesterol appears in the plasma, and so in the bile and faeces.

Amazingly, certain lipidiologists, dieticians, and institutions such as certain Heart Foundations (the latter in fact a public-orientated offshoot of the AHA) still persist today in all the above AHA recommendations, despite them showing little, if any, beneficial effect.

The Margarine Hoax

The magic words that initiated the margarine health conception were "Polyunsaturated fatty acids lower the blood cholesterol", derived from a short ten-months study in the USA. This was manna to the fledgeling margarine industry in the early 1960s. Their claims to have the highest polyunsaturated fatty acid content in their products was published, broadcast and televised throughout the world. A brilliant propaganda programme made them one of the richest food industries in the world.

However, with time it soon became clear that as a cholesterol-lowering and heart attack-lessening factor, results with margarine were not only disappointing and negative, but in fact proved the opposite. Claims were spread that the decline in deaths from heart attacks worldwide after 1963 were entirely due to this new life-saving product, totally ignoring the fact that 1963 was the year that emergency coronary units were introduced worldwide.

The "magic words" referred to above were incomplete. They should, more accurately, have stated that, "**Natural** polyunsaturated fatty acids lower the cholesterol, **but do not necessarily lessen heart attacks.**" All margarines contain many abnormal fatty acids which increase the blood cholesterol values.

Research is frequently carried out either as an experiment or as a study. An experiment is of short length, a few weeks to a few months. Studies are of a much longer period, at least four years, and can last up to 25 years or more. Studies look at the final endpoint, which, unfortunately in heart studies, is either heart attacks or deaths therefrom.

One experiment and four studies reported since 1990 have unequivocally indicated that margarine is harmful to health, and no other study has shown the opposite. Drs Mensink and Katan of the Netherlands placed 59 young adults on three different diets (10% energy intake provided as oleic acid, or as transoleic acid, or as saturated fat) for three weeks. Both the transoleic acid (as in margarine) and saturated fat increased the LDL-cholesterol values (*NEJM* 1990; 323: 439-45).

In the Caerphilly study in South Wales on men on a free-living diet, at the halfway mark in 1991, the results showed that, of 250 men on polyunsaturated margarine 9.6% had heart attacks, while of 1 380 men on butter only

5.3% had heart attacks. Furthermore it showed that the more full-cream milk that was drunk, the less the heart attacks; of 164 men who drank more than one pint of milk a day only 1.2% had heart attacks, and of 162 men who drank no milk 9.9% had heart attacks.

In a study on 85 095 women in the Nurses' Health Study in the USA over eight years, Dr Walter C. Willett and his co-workers from Boston Medical School reported that transfatty acids in margarine, cookies, cake and white bread increased both blood cholesterol and heart attacks (*Lancet* 1993; 341: 581-85).

In a case-control study of 239 persons admitted for a first heart attack in a Boston Hospital between 1 January 1982 and 31 December 1983, Dr Albert Ascherio and his co-workers showed that the intake of transfatty acids (as in margarine) led to an increase of heart attacks (*Circulation* 1994; 89: 94-101).

Furthermore, the famous Framingham Study, ongoing since 1948, near Harvard Medical School, has also indicated that the intake of margarine predisposes to heart attacks (35th Annual Conference on Cardiovascular Disease, 1995).

Most important is that four of these studies, Caerphilly, Ascherio, Nurses' Health Study and Framingham, all proved that the intake of butter was no risk for heart attacks. The reason is evident: butter has been a food for man universally for near enough 10 000 years, and man has become genetically adapted to it.

It is amazing how history repeats itself. Dr Bronte-Stewart of Cape Town reported in *The Lancet*, 1953, that hydrogenated fats (which are produced in margarine manufacture and are in fact abnormal transfatty acids) increases the blood cholesterol. Even Ancel Keys in the *Journal of Nutrition*, 1961, reported the same fact, adding that triglycerides and phospholipids were also increased.

The Margarine Propaganda Fightback

Little doubt exists from a scientific base that margarine in all its forms, tub or stick, soft, hard or polyunsaturated, has been proved harmful to man. The margarine industry and its scientific supporters, however, are not prepared to admit that their life's work has been incorrect and to no avail. They raise the following arguments.

"If the primary problem is transfatty acids, what about the transfatty acids in butter?" In the first place the primary problem is not transfatty acids but genetics. The latter will be discussed later.

The main harmful transfatty acid (TFA) in margarine is a monounsaturated TFA, elaidic acid. The total TFAs in margarine are 7-24% (*Lancet* 1993; 341: 581-85).

$H_3C\text{\\/\\/\\/}9\text{=/\\/\\/}COOH$ Transelaidic acid

The above has no receptor in human or animal metabolism.

The TFA in butter, transvaccinic acid, has been formed in the rumen of cows ever since cows produced milk. Consequently man has genetically adapted to it. However, fast-fed cows may contain abnormal TFAs in their milk through their commercial feeds, but the concentration of the latter is very low, 1-3%.

$H_3C\text{\\/\\/}11\text{=/\\/\\/}11\ COOH$ Transvaccinic acid

For the latter a receptor is present in human metabolism.

Abnormal TFAs cannot be taken up by the normal receptors for fatty acids, and therefore float around the body, especially in fat tissues, as foreign bodies with the danger of causing cancer.

Table 3.5 indicates the comparative butter/margarine consumption in different countries in the world during 1986 (*SAMJ* 1994; 84: 46-7).

The margarine lipidiologists argue, "that the TFAs are of lesser importance than the saturated fats, which are in higher concentration in butter, and increase the blood cholesterol". Ever since the Seven Countries Study, statements have been persistently made that saturated and animal fats increase the cholesterol. However, no mechanism has ever explained this supposed-to-be fact. Frequently such statements have had to be modified.

Average blood cholesterols have increased during Westernisation in many races, and the explanation has been that it is due to increased cholesterol intake in the diet. However, in a Westernised community a change in the cholesterol alone in the diet has led to only one out of seven persons (15%) showing a corresponding change in blood cholesterol ("Heart-Diet Study", *Circulation* 1986; 86: 759). Similar results were obtained in the very large Multiple Risk Factor Intervention Trial (MRFIT), 1985, and Lipid Research Clinics Coronary Prevention Trial (LRP-CPPT), 1984.

	Butter		Margarine	
	Kg/cap	%	Kg/cap	%
France	8.9	70.6	3.71	29.4
Switzerland	6.7	62.6	4.0	37.4
Irish Republic	6.7	61.6	4.2	38.4
Finland	7.9	55.5	7.2	44.5
Germany	8.8	50.0	7.9	50.0
Canada	3.99	42.4	5.43	57.6
Belgium	8.61	40.4	12.65	59.6
Austria	4.8	40.0	7.2	60.0
USA	4.6	39.2	11.2	60.8
UK	4.5	37.7	7.4	62.3
Sweden	7.1	34.9	3.22	65.1
Holland	3.6	31.6	11.4	68.4
Denmark	7.3	30.6	16.4	69.4
Iceland	5.4	30.3	12.1	69.7
Australia	3.8	30.0	8.9	70.0
Japan	0.7	26.3	1.96	73.7
Norway	4.2	23.7	13.3	76.3
South Africa	0.42	12.3	2.99	87.7

Table 3.5. Butter vs. margarine. Consumption kilograms per capita (Kg/cap.) and percentages for the year 1986 (South African Dairy Board, *SAMJ* 1994; 84: 46-7).

An important clue presents itself when lipidiologists state that "blood cholesterol increases especially when saturated fats are substituted for carbohydrates in the diet" (Schrapnell W.S. et al., *Med J Australia* 1992; 156: S9-S16). Carbohydrates have the highest micronutrient content. Little doubt exists that micronutrients lower blood cholesterol (De Villiers L.S., *Med Hypothesis* 1994; 42: 149-158). It is therefore reasonable to accept the fact that the **loss of micronutrients** in Western diets is the main factor in causing a raised blood cholesterol. Therefore it appears that only a non-causative association exists between a raised cholesterol and increased saturated fats.

A parallel comparison can be made between night darkness, a shining moon and a setting sun. A noncausative association exists between night darkness and a shining moon, but it is the causative association of a setting sun that causes the moon to shine (Fig 3.4).

In a further fight-back attempt much publicity was given to a New Zealand study (*BMJ* 1996; 312: 931-4) in which the authors claimed that "the use of unsaturated margarine rather than butter by persons with high cholesterols is associated with a lipogram profile that would be expected to reduce cardiovascular risk". With due respect, lipidiologists are better known for their expectations rather than their results. The facts are that the final endpoint, i.e. heart attacks or deaths therefrom, were in all studies much higher with margarine than with butter, where they were compared.

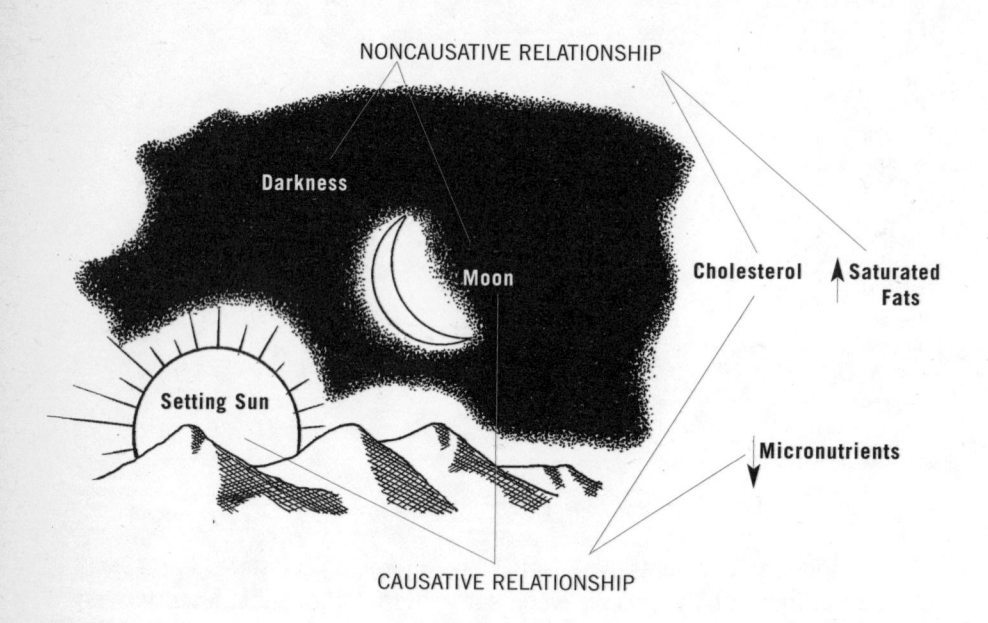

Fig 3.4. Causative vs. noncausative relationship. An illustration of the causative relationship between a) a setting sun and a shining moon, and b) an increase in cholesterol and a decrease in micronutrients, and a noncausative relationship between c) a shining moon and darkness and d) an increase in cholesterol and an increase in saturated fats.

A report on TFAs sponsored by the International Life Sciences Institute (*Am J Clin Nutr* 1995; 62: 655S-708S) is supported by the lipidiologists but criticised by the nutritionists. In a lengthy report it merely states that there is not enough evidence to condemn margarine, and in fact, only calls for further research. This is an old ruse of the lipidiologists in an attempt to delay the final admission that their life's work has been a failure.

The Role of Commerce

When the halfway results of the Caerphilly Study after five years were reported, they were so unexpected thanks to years of misleading propaganda, that a hastily convened Medical Research Council Panel advised that the Caerphilly findings should be ignored.

An immediate reaction was elicited from a large number of the medical profession. One, Dr W.W. Yellowlees of Aberfeldy, wrote a scathing critical letter to *The Lancet* (1991; 357: 1041-2). The following is an extract from it.

"Is not the attempt by the MRC panel to discredit the findings of the Cardiff Unit a good example of what Solzhenitsyn has called 'the censorship of fashion'? The fashionable teaching about dietary fats and heart disease could never have survived without widespead censorship of evidence against a theory, made popular by the evangelism of specialists and the interests of commerce."

CHAPTER 4

CORONARY HEART DISEASE: FACT OR FICTION

And as she looked around, she saw how Death, the consoler,
Laying his hand upon many a heart, had healed it forever.
LONGFELLOW, 1807-1882

Introduction

Henry Wadsworth Longfellow died two years after an unheralded historic event that was eventually to lead to the most devastating effect on man's health, the introduction of roller mills. Yet, at the time, the latter was hailed as a great breakthrough for the food industry. After thousands of years all grain foods were now "purified" and rid of all "impurities".

For the next century man was to enjoy his white bread, biscuits, cakes, white rice and white maize, yet all in the face of an alarming rising death rate, not only in heart disease, but in many other new or modern diseases, including cerebral accidents, diabetes and cancer. However, his physician would tell him that everything would be fine as long as he kept his daily cholesterol intake to below 300 mg, cut his animal fats to 10% of his daily energy values, increased his vegetable fats to 10% and kept his monounsaturated fats also at 10%. As the physician was a little vague on diets, he would refer his patient to a dietician.

All would be fine if he cut down or even excluded red meat, ate no more than two eggs per day, drank only milk containing 2% fat, excluded fatty cheeses, excluded butter and replaced it with polyunsaturated margarine, and added more vegetable oils to his foods. Most important, he had to bring his blood cholesterol down to below 5.2 mmol/l. If his diet failed to lower his cholesterol to this level, there were numerous drugs which would do the trick.

Even if he did have a heart attack, and was one of the lucky 60% to survive, there were always the emergency coronary units, established in all advanced countries, to control his heartbeat and thereby save his life. On the sidelines numerous surgeons were at hand, specifically trained to do bypass surgery on his heart, and so give him relief for a few more years.

From the 1970s on he was told to eat more roughage, more fibre, wholewheat bread rather than white, brown rice in preference to white rice; to eat more unrefined maize if it was available, sprinkle his food with digestive bran, eat more of large leaf vegetables, and partake of more fresh fruit. Instructions on fats, however, were to be even more strict than ever before.

Yet modern man's thoughts went back to the dietary pattern of his grandparents and great-grandparents. They ate all the foods now prohibited for heart disease, yet few if any of them had heart attacks, and they frequently reached a ripe old age. On questioning their physicians on these facts, the latter would explain, after considerable hesitation, that the persons of those times had more exercise and less worries. Neither the patients nor the physicians were convinced by these explanations.

Lipids and Atherosclerosis

The work of the Russians Anitschkow and Chalatow in 1913 has already been mentioned. They are regarded as the fathers of the lipid theory. Although their opinions stimulated interest, it was limited interest, since deaths from heart attacks were then still extremely rare.

A Dutch physician De Lange, in 1916, related high blood cholesterols to increased incidences of atherosclerosis in Javanese stewards working aboard Dutch ships. He also noted that atherosclerosis was rare among native Javanese. These latter facts are important when we relate it to high cholesterol diets.

Towards the end of the 1920s it was noted that deaths from heart attacks had suddenly begun increasing. This prompted the decision to initiate a separate list of deaths from heart attacks in the *International List of Causes of Death*, as metioned in Chapter 2. The figure in 1929 in the USA was 25.7 per 100 000 population, and only 34 years later in 1963 it reached its peak at 307 per 100 000, a staggering twelvefold increase within 34 years. In this short period it had become the number one killer in all Westernised countries.

Heart attacks now became the number one priority in medicine. Amongst the enthusiasts was Dr Ancel Keys of Minnesota, Minneapolis, primary a physiologist, but later an epidemiologist and nutritionist. An enthusiastic and dynamic person, he persuaded his colleagues in Europe and Japan to join him in the Seven Countries Study to ascertain the role of fats in heart disease. Unfortunately, his preoccupation with fats led to the disputed findings that polyunsaturated and vegetable fats got the go-ahead, while saturated and animal fats were considered the guilty party. Primarily Keys never blamed dietary cholesterol, but was apparently later persuaded to this opinion by his colleagues and co-workers.

A group of contemporary researchers strongly questioned the results of the Seven Countries Study. One, Yerushalmy, noted that if the proteins had been considered they would also have been shown as being important factors in heart disease (*N Y State J of Medicine*, 1957). But Ancel Keys, a prolific writer, dynamic speaker and worldwide traveller, was not to be denied, and he stuck to his guns, now loaded with fats.

The number of lipid researchers now increased phenomenally, for here, it was believed, lay the answer to defeating our biggest killer. New lipid journals sprung into being and lipid articles appeared by the thousands. All Heart Associations, especially in America, endorsed the lipid theory and played a leading role in advising the public. Their dietary advice has already been discussed in the previous chapter.

Low-Density and High-Density Lipoprotein-Cholesterols (LDL, HDL) and Triglycerides

Total cholesterol can be subdivided into various fractions, the two most important being LDL- and HDL-cholesterols. These two differ according to the density (solidity, consistency) of their constituents. Proteins are far heavier and more dense than fats (Table 4.1.).

In simple terms, the functions of these two lipoproteins differ in that LDL carries cholesterol to the peripheral tissues where it is released to perform its important functions, whereas HDL carries cholesterol away from the peripheral tissues back to the liver. Here some of the cholesterol again joins the pathway to the tissues, but a large portion is freed and eventually excreted in the bile and faeces (Fig 4.1). Consequently LDL has become known as the **bad** cholesterol and HDL as the **good** cholesterol.

How bad and how good will be shown later. The ratio of LDL:HDL in the blood is normally 4:1 in man. In nonmeat-eating animals, such as antelopes, the ratio is 1:1.

From a risk factor point of view a high LDL and a low HDL are considered high-risk factors for heart disease, as would a high LDL:HDL ratio. However it is now becoming recognised that a rise in HDL is a protective action secondary to a rise in LDL. It is when this mechanism fails that the risk of heart attacks appears to increase.

On the other hand, in primitive races that have not come into contact with

	PROTEIN	PHOSPHO-LIPIDS	FREE CHOL.	CHOL. ESTERS	TRIGLYC-ERIDES
LDL	20	20	18	36	8
HDL	45	30	8	18	0

In percentages.

Table 4.1. The concentrations and physio-chemical illustrations of LDL- and HDL-cholesterol.

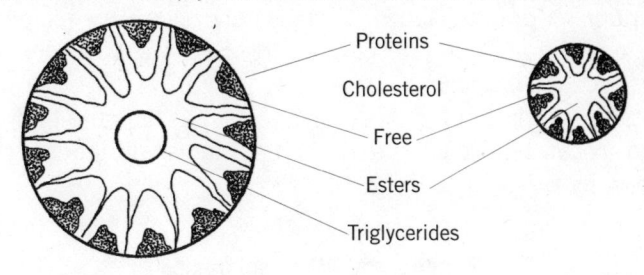

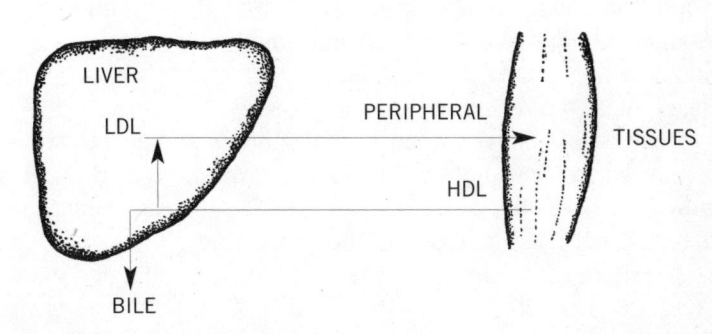

Fig 4.1. The metabolism of LDL- and HDL-cholesterol.

foods unnatural to their genetic diets, both LDL and HDL are low. Nature is therefore responsible for both low LDLs and HDLs.

In many of the studies on heart attacks which are limited to blood lipid investigations, HDL is frequently the only significant risk factor in marginal statistical results.

Of great significance is the presence of **cholesterol esters** in both LDL and HDL. Esters are combinations containing fatty acids. The fact that approximately 85% of these fatty acid concentrations are under control of micronutrients for their metabolism, is probably the most important key to the role of cholesterol in atherosclerosis. This will be discussed fully later.

Triglycerides consist of three fatty acids in combination with glycerol. In absorption of fat by the gut, fatty acids are the earliest absorbed, causing turbidity or cloudiness of the blood. Numerous studies on triglycerides in atherosclerosis have indicated a weak correlation with heart disease. However, it does appear that diabetics are unable to metabolise triglycerides sufficiently. Consequently the two most common conditions increasing blood triglycerides are diabetes and the aftereffects of fatty meals. Fasting 12 to 14 hours prior to drawing blood is absolutely necessary for an accurate triglyceride estimation. A number of rare congenital diseases can cause gross hypertriglyceridaemia, appearing as a milky serum.

As at least one or two of the three fatty acids that form the triglyceride are unsaturated, it can be expected that micronutrients will lower triglycerides, as was shown by Brusis in 1986.

Proteins and Atherosclerosis

Ignatowski's protein theory had, however, not been forgotten. In 1925 Drs Newburgh and Marsh of Michigan, USA, initiated an experiment in which the then known amino acids were fed individually to animals in an attempt to establish which amino acids could be responsible for the atherosclerotic changes. Alas, the results were all negative.

In those days, however, international communication was still in its infancy. Unknown to Newburgh and Marsh, a new amino acid had been discovered by Dr J.H. Muller of Germany in 1922. This was **methionine** which, of course, had not been included in the above study.

The next clue came in 1930 when a child aged eight and mentally retarded, developed severe atherosclerosis, and died shortly afterwards from a heart attack. The cause of this early onset of atherosclerosis could at that time not be established.

In 1932 De Vigneaue discovered a substance, **homocysteine**, formed from methionine.

World War II followed, bringing not only advances in warfare, but also in medicine. Added vitamins in troops' rations had a surprisingly good effect on their general health. In 1949 Drs Rhinehart and Greenberg, USA, initiated an experiment in which the results of single vitamin deficiencies in rhesus monkeys were investigated. Vitamin B6 depletion in the diet showed little general effect externally, but the researchers were surprised to discover a considerable local effect on the blood vessels with advanced general atherosclerosis.

In 1962 two siblings with advanced atherosclerosis were discovered by Drs Carlson and Neill. More cases with similar findings and related to the 1930 children were also discovered. Due to medical research advances, the cause could now be established. A high concentration of homocysteine was discovered in the blood and urine. This is a normal product of methionine, the amino acid missing from Newburgh and Marsh's experiments. The cause of the increase in homocysteine in these children was an enzyme fault, **cystathionine synthase**, which caused the raised blood homocysteine (Fig 4.2). This is a true genetic fault known as homocystinuria, which was later established as present in about one in 50 000 to one in 100 000 persons.

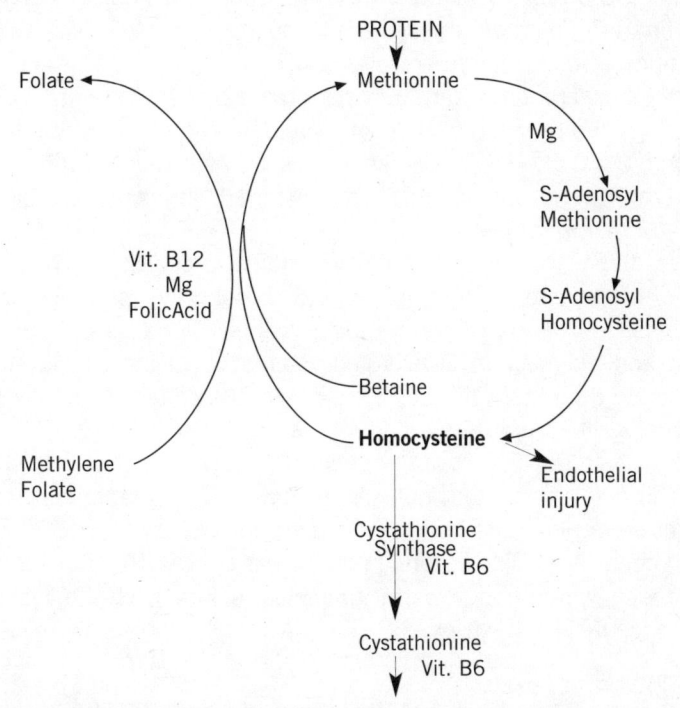

Fig 4.2. The homocysteine metabolism. Note the roles of the four micronutrients, vitamin B6, folic acid, vitamin B12 and magnesium. Note the position of the enzyme, cystathionine synthase, which when genetically decreased or absent causes homocystinuria.

Amongst the researchers who investigated the children with homocystinuria was a pathologist from New York, Dr Kilmer McCully. A brilliant scientist, he now gave thought to a number of indicators that could suggest an alternative to the lipid theory for atherosclerosis. These included the following:

1. Ignatowski's protein theory.
2. The discovery of methionine in 1922, the amino acid that was excluded in Newburgh and Marsh's experiments in 1925.
3. Methionine as the forerunner of homocysteine in metabolism.
4. Rhinehart and Greenberg's experiments with the exclusion of Vitamin B6 in the diet leading to atherosclerosis.
5. The appearance of the hereditary disease, homocystinuria, with widespread atherosclerosis.

Could homocysteine, which had not been considered of any particular importance until the discovery of the congenital condition homocystinuria, be a possible link in human atherosclerosis? Would a slight to reasonable rise in homocysteine also lead to atherosclerosis?

Numerous experiments were now performed on various animals: rabbits, baboons, pigs and rats, in which a solution of homocysteine was infused into their blood (McCully 1970; Harker, Ross 1974; Reddy 1982). Without exception all these experiments demonstrated the same pathology: an increase in atherosclerosis.

In 1975 McCully reported his theory: atherosclerosis can be caused by an increase of homocysteine in the blood, due to not only a shortage of vitamin B6, but also, as a result of further experiments, shortages of vitamin B12, folic acid and magnesium. The homocysteine acted as a toxic substance which irritated the inner layers of the arteries, the endothelium, causing the endothelium cells to proliferate and increase.

Two large problems, however, kept the homocysteine theory in the background. The first was the difficulty in establishing a reliable method for its quantification in blood, its normal concentration being only 1/500th of normal blood cholesterol. The second problem was the terrific preponderance of the lipid theory which had powerful financial backing from the vegetable-oil and pharmaceutical industries.

The Heart Study that Shocked the World

Shortly after the Korean War started in 1950, the Pentagon in the USA sent pathologists to the combat zone to examine wound ballistics. However, these wise doctors, while doing autopsies, noticed some unexpected findings in the young soldiers' arteries. The average age of these soldiers was only 22 years, yet signs of atherosclerosis were already present.

Wisely, they decided to examine 300 consecutive cases in which they methodologically investigated the coronary arteries of the heart. Two pathological pictures were represented. In 35% they discovered streaks of fat and fibre deposits, the fatty streak already the earliest sign of atherosclerosis. But worse than that, 42% showed the more advanced hard fibrous plaques, including cholesterol deposits, dead tissue and calcium. The latter was similar to the picture seen in advanced atherosclerosis, a condition which was believed to develop only in 40- to 50-year-olds. Of these young men in the youthful prime of their lives, 77% showed danger signs of approaching heart disease.

With the death rate from this disease rapidly rising to the top of the list, the medical world now realised that drastic steps must be taken immediately to find a solution. Studies on human populations were necessary, unfortunately necessitating many years' delay in finding a solution. But there was no alternative.

The Major Heart Studies

It is common sense that the more persons volunteering to take part in a study, the more reliable the results. But then the more taking part, the higher the costs.

One study had already been initiated in 1948. A team from Boston University Medical School undertook to investigate a portion of the adult population of an industrial town, **Framingham**, eighteen miles west of Boston. Of this population of 28 000 inhabitants, eventually 5 127 healthy men and women were to be investigated for the rest of their lives. Initially this study was helpful in establishing a number of risk factors for heart disease – an increase in age, high blood pressure, smoking, obesity, a sedentary lifestyle and a high blood cholesterol. Men were more prone than women, premenopausal women were practically immune.

The Framingham Study is still continuing, and in the last few years has reported some surprising and important results. These will be discussed later.

The second major study was the **Multiple Risk Factor Intervention Trial** (MRFIT), initiated in 1973, in which 361 662 middle-aged men were investigated for the role of three known risk factors, smoking, high blood pressure and high blood cholesterol. Of these persons 12 866 candidates at high risk were chosen. They were divided into two groups; the one would receive "special attention" from highly trained personnel to control their diet, cut down on their smoking and treat their blood pressure. The other group would receive "routine treatment" from their own physicians. The study would last seven years.

To say the least, the results were disappointing. There were no significant differences in the number of deaths from heart attacks between the two groups, despite the fact that the special attention group decreased their cholesterol intake by 40%, saturated fat by 28% and total calories by 21%. Furthermore the average blood cholesterol values only decreased by 5% instead of the expected 10%. (NB: This points to a genetic factor controlling the blood cholesterol.)

The third major study was the **Coronary Primary Prevention Trial** (CPPT). Here a well-planned experiment, encompassing twelve major research centres in the USA, would attempt to see what effect a cholesterol-lowering drug would have on lessening the death rate from heart attacks. Out of 480 000 middle-aged men 3 810 with blood cholesterols above 6.85 mmol/l (265 mg%), the top 5% of cholesterol values, were to be divided into two groups. The one group would receive the drug cholestyramine, which would interfere with the absorption of cholesterol by binding it with bile. The other group would receive a placebo which looks and tastes the same as the real drug but has no effect. The trial would be double-blind, i.e. neither the volunteers nor the investigators would know who received the drug and who the placebo. It would be the most expensive study yet, 142 million dollars (*JAMA* 1984; 251: 351-374).

In January 1984 the results of the CPPT were announced with much fanfare. The journal *Time*, 23 January 1984, had the following headlines on the cover and inside, "Sorry, it's True. Cholesterol really is a killer! No whole milk. No butter. No fatty meats. Fewer eggs". One of the supposed "messages" that came out of the study and is still widely reported at present, is that "for every 1% reduction in serum cholesterol a 2% reduction in heart attacks would follow". Even if this were true, it must be remembered that it would only apply to the 5% of the population with blood cholesterols above 6.85 mmol/l (265 mg%).

The fourth major study was the **Helsinki Heart Study** where 4 081 men, 40 to 55 years of age, were divided into two groups, one receiving Gemfibrosil (Lopid) which decreased the absorption of cholesterol, while the other group received a placebo (*NEJM* 1987; 317: 1237-46). Statistically only the increase in HDL-cholesterol was the strongest prediction of a reduction in heart attacks.

A bitter controversy developed over the interpretation of these and other heart studies. The lipidiologists declared, "Yes, cholesterol could be lowered, leading to a lowering of heart-death rates. Yes, the lowering of particularly the LDL-cholesterol was of more importance than total cholesterol. The importance of raising the HDL-cholesterol was the most decisive result, correlating well with a lowering of the death rate."

A large body of prominent cardiologists and nutritionists, however, did not agree. "The changes were insignificant. The application of biased statistics exaggerated minor gains and underplayed negative results." There was even talk of data torturing.

"If you torture your data long enough, it will tell you whatever you want it to tell" (*NEJM* 1993; 329: 1196-9).

The Cholesterol Strategists

It is said that if you wish to stress a weak point, bark loud like a dog, growl menacingly like a lion, then run swiftly away like a jackal. The lipidiologists appointed a carefully selected panel of fourteen lipid researchers, nominated by the National Heart, Lung and Blood Institute of the USA, at the end of 1984 to organise a "Consensus Development Congress" with its main concern the role of cholesterol in heart disease. Any "consensus congress" is notorious for limiting "voters" to participants with predetermined similar views, but astutely inviting a wide spectrum of interested experts with no right to vote.

The main presenter at this "congress" was Dr Basil Rifkind, the director of the CPP Trial. His main theme would be the "conclusive" results of the latter trial. This was followed by recommendations on diet, which were similar if not identical to the American Heart Association's so-called "prudent" diet.

For two days speaker after speaker from the floor argued and warned against the overemphasis of cholesterol importance, as well as of the diet supposed to lower blood cholesterol. However, when it came to the final report, as drawn up by the chosen panel, it was clear that they were set on their own views, and the opinions of the nonpanel debaters were to be ignored. The panel decided that it had been established "beyond reasonable doubt" that lowering of the elevated cholesterol levels, especially of LDL-cholesterol, would reduce the risks of heart attacks. Furthermore, the average levels of Americans' blood cholesterol levels were too high due to "the high dietary intake of calories, saturated fat and cholesterol". They knew they would have the moral and financial backing of two powerful industries, the pharmaceutical and vegetable fat industries.

An immediate reaction was provoked in many researchers, who were shocked at the Consensus Meeting's report. The first two to react, both present at the meeting were Prof Edward Ahrens of Rockefeller University, and

Prof Michael Oliver of Edinburgh University, who, in two successive articles in *The Lancet*, condemned the one-sided and poorly substantiated advice of the panel, which quoted studies with minimum or even negative results. Prof Oliver wrote of the "non-sensus of consensus".

The Cholesterol-Education Programme of the AHA

If you cannot hammer a nail through a piece of wood, just keep on hammering; it may make some impression. To the shock of the lipidiologists they discovered that although the majority of the public believed their propaganda, the majority of the physicians did not agree with them. Only 28% of the physicians thought a high-fat diet could lead to heart attacks, and only 39% believed a high blood cholesterol was a heart attack risk (*JAMA* 1987; 258: 3521). The physicians could speak from personal experience.

It was therefore imperative that the propaganda directed at the public should now be broadened to include the medical profession, so they argued. But the latter wanted something more than just subjective opinions.

Once more the National Heart, Lung and Blood Institute sponsored a group known as the National Cholesterol Education Programme (NCEP) with the primary goal of influencing the physician community in favour of lowering blood cholesterol and applying its proposed cholesterol-lowering diet. Much to the Institute's disappointment, the approval to go ahead with the programme was only reached after three meetings over six-months periods each. The appointed panel had twice refused to endorse the chairman's proposals.

It is important to emphasise that the decision to which the panel now came was purely an arbitrary one, i.e. with no proof and with no previous experience, no better than guesswork and speculation.

Normal values of laboratory biochemical tests have traditionally always been determined by measuring blood values of at least 120 normal persons, and then deleting the top and bottom 5%. This was called the normal range 90%. It applied to glucose, uric acid, urea and a hundred other blood constituents, including cholesterol.

However, interpreting blood cholesterol levels in the above manner hampered the lipidiologists in their theories. The majority of the panel members decided that new normal values were to be applied to cholesterol, more acceptable to the cholesterol theory.

The best suited would be if the 40th percentile (at the 40% mark of the values) would distinguish between the "desirable" values, and the "lower risk" cases, while the 75th percentile (at the 75% mark of the values) would distinguish between the "low risk" and the "high risk" cases. The

CORONARY HEART DISEASE: FACT OR FICTION • 69

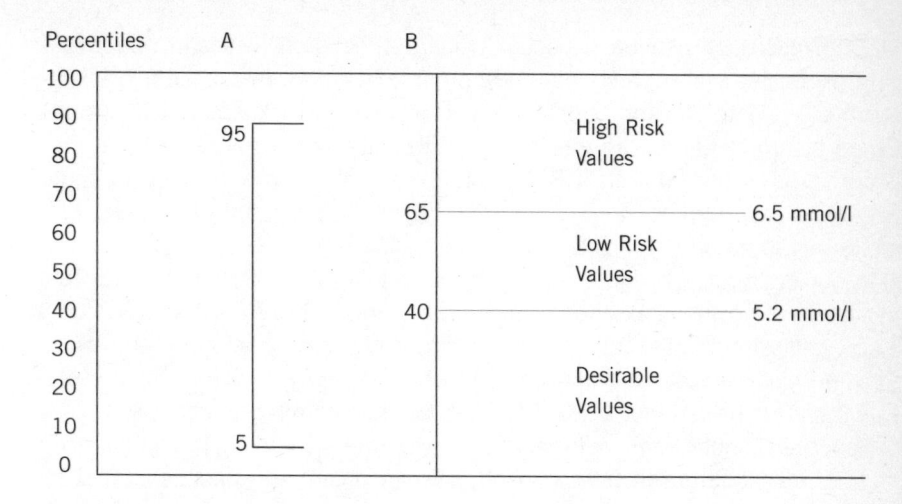

Fig 4.3. Recommendations for blood cholesterol interpretations comparing those of the National Cholesterol Education Programme (B, 1988) with those of traditional methods (A, Normal values 90%). Percentiles indicate the percentage of persons with those values.

40th percentile coincided with the 5.2 mmol/l (200 mg%) value, and the 75th percentile with the 6.5 mmol/l (250 mg%) value (*Arch Int Med* 1988; 148: 36-69) (Fig 4.3).

Let it again be stressed, this was an arbitrary decision with no experimental proof whatsoever. In other words, at its best it was a guess based on studies which were only fractionally suggestive of meaning, and others that were not.

But you cannot classify without advice for treatment. The "high risk" cases would require medical treatment for the rest of their lives. The "low risk" cases would require medical treatment with one additional risk factor in men, and with two additional risk factors in women. These additional risk factors included high blood pressure, family history of heart disease, obesity, diabetes, smoking, low levels of HDL and other blood vessel diseases. As invariably one or more of the latter are present in these patients, all would have to receive treatment.

Those with values below 5.2 mmol/l were to be provided with brochures on cholesterol and to be retested after five years.

How Accurate Are Cholesterol Estimations?

This is an exceedingly important question if the above values are to be considered. The majority of patients are placed in mortal fear of their cholesterol values falling in the "danger group", and await their results with trepidation.

High accuracy can be expected from a specialised research laboratory with expensive and sophisticated equipment. However, by far the majority of routine cholesterol estimations are performed in commercial laboratories where accuracy cannot be guaranteed. Even in the specialised laboratories accuracy is accepted with a 3% error, i.e. a 5.0 mmol/l cholesterol could record values from 4.85 to 5.15 mmol/l, while a 6.0 mmol/l cholesterol could record values from 5.82 to 6.18 mmol/l.

A survey by the College of American Pathologists found that the error rate in a group of private laboratories erred by an average of 6.2%, i.e. a 5.0 mmol/l blood cholesterol could record values from 4.69 to 5.31 mmol/l, and a 6.0 mmol/l blood cholesterol could vary from 5.63 to 6.37 mmol/l. Still worse, a 1988 survey showed that 20% of laboratories had an error rate of 9%, i.e. a 5 mmol/l blood cholesterol could vary from 4.63 to 5.45 mmol/l.The author once had 30 ml blood drawn from himself, divided it into six specimens of 5 ml each, and sent one to each of six different local laboratories. The head of each laboratory was personally phoned and informed of the steps taken, and was requested to give special to attention to accuracy. The results received were 3.9, 4.2, 4.8, 5.2, 5.6, and 5.8 mmol/l, with each laboratory adamant that their estimation was as accurate as could be.

A similar experience was reported by Walt Bogdarich, a *Wall Street Journal* reporter. He sent blood samples to five different laboratories in New York. Results returned placed him in the high risk, low risk and borderline groups. A Pulitzer Prize winner, he published these results in the *Wall Street Journal* of 2-3 February 1987.

LDL-cholesterol and HDL-cholesterol values are even more difficult to determine accurately, due to their lower concentrations. Yet significant interpretations are accorded variations in these values. The use of inexpensive desk-top apparatus for cholesterol estimations is extremely inaccurate, even with expensive control fluids.

Different international and national quality control systems are universally available for laboratories to verify their results, but participation is not enforced. With numerous of these systems present, who is to determine which system is the most accurate?

These inaccuracies should have been known to the Cholesterol Education Programme panelists, yet they persisted in declaring precise cut-off values. It would have been wise to declare certain grey areas. At least it would have had the effect of partly allaying some of the personal fears of a large proportion of the public as to their cholesterol value interpretations.

Criticism of the Primary Cholesterol Theory as well as the Advice on Diet

Although the cholesterol-lipid theory had its fault-finders from its inception with Anitschkow's findings in 1913, the criticism reached a peak during the 1980s. This came primarily from renowned researchers in the field of cardiology, nutrition and epidemiology, but also from certain thinkers and observers in general practice. Few critics would argue that cholesterol and lipids played no role, but it had all to be put into perspective. The strategy of emphasising minor positive results and ignoring negative ones was to be deplored.

Past president of the British Cardiac Society, Michael Oliver of Edinburgh and London, repeats his arguments that the death rate had not been reduced in any of the studies in which blood cholesterol was lowered (*J Am Coll Cardiology*, Sept 1988). Exceptions to the above rule were two studies applying nicotinic acid. The latter is a vitamin with at least 420 functions as a cofactor to enzymes, including control of the important prostaglandin balance.

Eliot Corday, a physician, in the same journal, February 1989, records many reasons why American doctors have concerns about the "cholesterol-awareness programmes". He emphasises that it is only a small group of lipidiologists who are pushing the cholesterol theory, and describes it as "an unscientific approach that may cause the medical profession much harm and loss of respect in the future".

Gunning Scheepers in a leading article in *The Lancet*, 4 March 1989, states: "Future generations may look back upon the era of population interventions, as a means of prevention of cardiovascular diseases, with disbelief and contempt for the epidemiological analysis that supported those political decisions."

Harsh words, but are they not undeniably true?

Dr Allan Brett in a leading article in the *New England Journal of Medicine*, 7 September 1989, agrees with Corday that the manner of reporting results by researchers has been misleading, and in fact dishonest. As examples he cites the two major studies, the CPPT and Helsinki Studies. The researchers limited the reporting of their results to a comparison between the number of heart attacks in treated and untreated (placebo) cases, with impressive sounding 19% and 33% differences respectively, so-called **relative** statistics. To give full meaning to their results they should have compared both total groups, not only those who had heart attacks. Now these **absolute** differences drop dramatically to 1.7% and 1.4% respectively, differences which are of little if any importance. The final differences are so small that Brett asks the question, "How, for example, does a 30-year-old man weigh the importance of an extra month of life in his 75th year?"

Brett's article and similar criticisms were brought to the public's attention in the *Reader's Digest* of September 1990, under the title, "New Questions about Cholesterol".

A book written by three prominent American researchers, *Balanced Nutrition: Beyond the Cholesterol Scare*, Stare, Olsen and Whelan, publishers Bob Adams, 1989, also severely criticises the cholesterol emphasis. They are all members of the powerful nonprofit-making American Council of Science and Health, of which Dr Elizabeth Whelan is a past president. Their booklet *The Facts and Myths about Coronary Heart Disease: A Consumer Guide* has gained wide recognition in the USA.

Prof Michael DeBakey, the famous pioneer heart surgeon who dissected and investigated every blood vessel he operated upon, found little correlation between blood cholesterol values and atherosclerosis. A personal letter from him to the author confirms this view, and he has been highly critical of the emphasis on fats as a cause of atherosclerosis.

Editorials in journals reflect the opinions of either the editor or of invited authorities on medical matters in which items of related importance are discussed. Since the campaign against fats and cholesterol was intensified from approximately 1985 onwards, a barrage of editorials from leading world medical journals have criticised the biased interpretations of the lipid researchers, warning against an oversimplification of the cholesterol-atherosclerosis issue. All have concluded that cholesterol has a role in atherosclerosis, but all agree that there is a lot more than just cholesterol that is important.

Dr Tunstall-Pedoe of Scotland notes the laughable situation where 84% of Scots men aged 55-64 yrs have blood cholesterols above 5.2 mmol/l, indicating low plus high risks, while 95% of Scots women of the same age have values over 5.2 mmol/l. Certain Scandinavian countries report similar findings. This makes a mockery of the Cholesterol Education Programme.

An Upsurge of Heart Surgery

Despite the publicity accorded the CEP and the low cholesterol-fat diet, little substantial progress was to be seen in fighting heart disease. The sharp decline in cardiac deaths after 1963 was accompanied by a 12% increase in cancers, especially prostate cancer in men and breast cancer in women (*NEJM* 1995; 332: 1491-98). However, in the rare cases where statistics for total heart attacks are available, deaths plus nondeaths, two studies showed a remarkable increase. In one study an 80% increase in heart attacks and 150% increase in costs of morbidity between 1977 and 1987 was recorded. In addition the famous Framingham Study had shown a steady increase in total heart attacks up to present times (*Lancet* 1993; 342: 977).

From the discerning public's point of view, a general scepticism developed due to the disappointment that so little had been achieved in heart disease cures. It was now the turn of the heart surgeons to move in. Two major heart surgery procedures became the fashion.

Prior to any surgery a thorough examination of the coronary arteries is required. This is obtained by coronary arteriography, which shows up details of the coronary arteries by injecting radio-opaque material into the blood (Fig 4.4).

One of the surgical procedures is coronary artery bypass surgery (CABS) in which a segment of an artery or a vein in the chest wall or from the leg is dissected, removed and used to cause a bypass or short cut from the aorta to pass the obstruction in the coronary arteries. The second procedure is percutaneous transluminal coronary angioplasty (PTCA), in which the cardiologist guides a

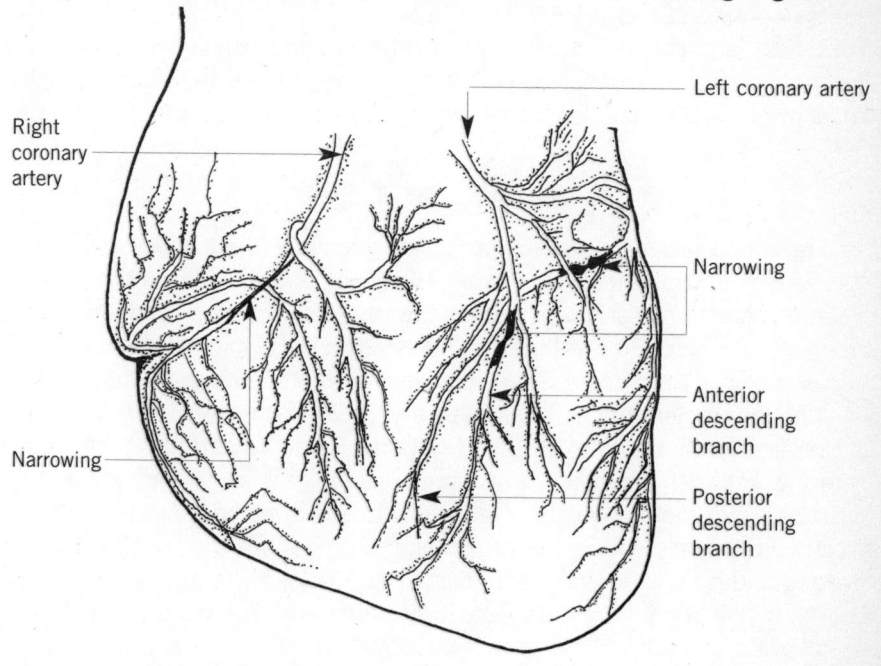

Fig 4.4. Coronary angiography. In coronary artherosclerosis the major arteries narrow or clots (thrombi) form, causing a heart attack or coronary thrombosis. The X-ray photo is taken after injecting a radiopaque substance intravenously.

small flexible balloon-capped catheter into the affected narrow coronary artery under X-ray, and in the narrowed area the balloon is inflated to widen the artery at that point.

The latter procedure (PTCA) is less stressful, but the return of the original lesion, known as restinosis, occurs within months in 30% to 40% of cases. CABS is a far more severe procedure, with 5 to 10% again closing within the first two weeks, and another 5 to 10% closing within the first year. For the rest, after a year in all cases, the atherosclerosis progresses inevitably (*NEJM* 1995; 332: 1491-8). In good hands surgical mortality in CABS is 1%, but it can be much higher in less able hands.

The problem is to prevent the return of progressive atherosclerosis. However, if this could be prevented, surgery would not be necessary in the first place. It is insufficiently appreciated that the traditional "known" risk factors explain only a proportion of the causes of coronary heart disease. Some authorities report only 50% (*BMJ* 1990; 301: 1004-5), while others report this figure as low as 28-42% (*Lancet* 1994; 343: 75-9).

It has been stated that on reinvestigation by independent experts of the presurgical findings in many cases of heart surgery in the USA, it was found that in as much as 50% of these cases surgery had been unnecessary.

The Importance of Aspirin

At a recent congress of physicians a speaker asked the question how many present partook of aspirin regularly. Two-thirds of the audience raised their hands. Then he asked who partook of micronutrients regularly. Again two-thirds raised their hands. Possibly it was the same two-thirds. How come the pharmaceutical industry places so much accent on aspirin and so little on micronutrients?

A major problem in cardiovascular disease is blood coagulation or thrombosis, frequently the final episode in the run-up to a heart attack. Aspirin's effect is to lower the chances of thrombosis. But most doctors and all laymen have a somewhat vague idea as how this is affected. "Aspirin decreases the prostaglandins", is the usual comment. But over 50 members of the prostaglandin family exist. Are all decreased?

The explanation – and note how it interlinks with the micronutrients – is as follows:.

Blood vessel constriction and aggregation of clumping of blood platelets depends upon a delicate balance between two eics, thomboxane A2 (TXA2) and prostaglandin I2 (PGI2). Aspirin inhibits or suppresses an enzyme, oxygenase, in blood platelets, which leads to a reduced formation of TXA2. The

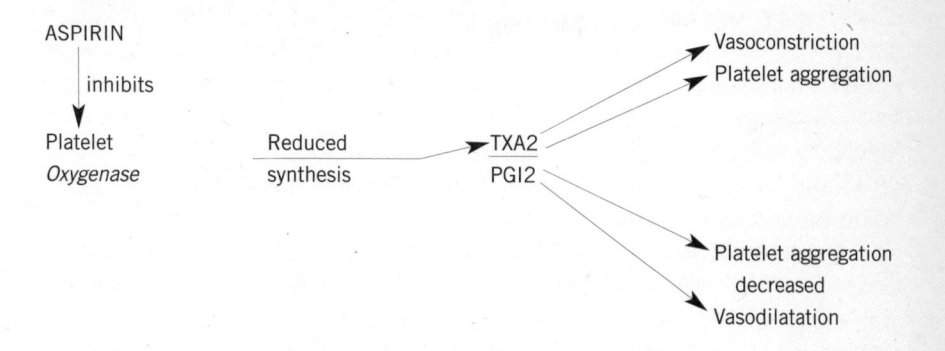

```
ASPIRIN                                              Vasoconstriction
                                                     Platelet aggregation
  | inhibits
  ▼
Platelet         Reduced         TXA2
Oxygenase        synthesis       PGI2

                                                     Platelet aggregation
                                                        decreased
                                                     Vasodilatation
```

Fig 4.5. The action of aspirin in decreasing platelet aggregation and increasing vasodilation, thereby decreasing the danger of a heart attack. Micronutrients do the same by normalising TXA2 and PGI2.

result is that the blood vessels dilate (expand) and the clumping of platelets decreases, thereby lessening the danger of a heart attack (*Eucasanoids* 1989; 2: 193-7) (See Fig 4.5).

But micronutrients do exactly the same and have been doing this for thousands of years.

Aspirin reduces nonfatal heart attacks and strokes by one-third, while deaths from these conditions are reduced by one-sixth. A half-tablet (160 mg) a day is considered sufficient. It is also used routinely after any of the heart blood vessel procedures, as well as in deep venous thrombosis (blood clots in the veins of the legs and elsewhere). However, the biggest risk factor for deep venous thrombosis appears to be increased blood homocysteine, which is well controlled by micronutrients.

There are certain dangers in aspirin therapy. It could lead to bleeding somewhere in the vicinity of blood vessels, and to irritation of the stomach lining. Micronutrients have none of these disadvantages.

The Nurses' Health Study had an interesting item on aspirin. It substantially reduced the risk of colon-rectal cancer (*NEJM* 1995; 333: 609-14), a finding only becoming apparent after 10 years of regular use. Micronutrients are known to be extremely effective against cancer.

Regular use of aspirin is said to be an inexpensive method of fighting heart disease, thrombosis and cancer. Alternatively micronutrients are far more effective in fighting the above diseases, are even less expensive, have a good effect on all modern metabolic diseases, increase the patient's general wellbeing, and have no complications or side effects.

What aspirins can do, micronutrients can do better.

Mediterranean Diets

Of all the developed areas in the world it appears that the inhabitants of the Mediterranean countries are the healthiest from a heart disease point of view, or at least that was so in the 1960s. Suggestions have been made that we should exclusively follow the Mediterranean diet and our heart problems would become something of the past.

The writings of Homer, the Greek poet who lived in 700 B.C., suggest that food in his time was almost exclusively meat, served with liberal quantities of bread and wine. Vegetables and fruits were rare.

A survey of diet comparing Crete, Greece and the USA for 1948-1949, is shown in Table 4.2 (*Am J Clin Nutr* 1995; 61: 1313S).

	CRETE %Energy	GREECE %Energy	USA %Energy
Cereals	39	61	25
Pulses, nuts, potatoes	11	8	6
Vegetables, fruits	11	5	6
Meat, fish, eggs	4	3	19
Dairy products	3	4	14
Table oils and fats	29	15	15
Sugar and honey	2	4	15
Wine, beer, spirits	1	*	*

* no data available

Table 4.2. A comparison of diets, 1948-1949 (*Am J Clin Nutr* 1995; 61: 1313S).

One particularly important diet factor which has received much publicity lately is olive oil. In Crete 78% of table fats are derived from this. Suggestions have been made that olive oil is the outstanding health factor in the Mediterranean diet. That may be, but it must also be realised that it is part of the genetic diet of those countries, being a dietary ingredient for thousands of years. If other genetic races should adopt olive oil as a basic factor in their diets, what certainty exists that metabolic diseases will not be generated due to this "foreign" foodstuff? It has happened before, e.g. margarine, and it could happen again.

But alas, even the inhabitants of these idyllic countries are doomed. They are fast changing their diets for the more palatable, if more micronutrient divested diets of a changing world. It has been suggested that Mediterranean diets may be becoming an endangered species.

The middle 1990s may in the future become known in the atherosclerosis world as the era of great decisions, when the two great theories reached a climax by discovering certain areas of agreement, while discarding vast areas of diversity or disagreement. These two theories are the lipid-cholesterol theory which will have to shed much, and the homocysteine-protaglandin-micronutrient theory, which will have to compromise on certain smaller aspects. Should these compromises be accepted, the world of medicine could settle for a final total viable theory in which micronutrients and genetics play a central role, encompassing homocysteine plus cholesterol in all its forms.

The Homocysteine Theory

Modern medical literature leaves the world in no doubt that at present an explosion on homocysteine research and theory is apparent. And yet few if any laymen in the street have ever heard the term. It should be more universal than "cholesterol", for it is eight times more of a risk factor in heart disease. It is as if the public media, which has so long exalted the importance of cholesterol, is unwilling to recognise any other killer in heart disease. If you tell a lie long enough you will eventually become conditioned to believe it. And no one wishes to admit to a lie, especially not a media man.

It would be impossible to summarise all the hundreds, perhaps thousands of articles now appearing on the role of homocysteine in atherosclerosis. Hardly a single leading international medical journal, especially in the field of nutrition, does not have some form of reference to its importance every week or month. All concur on the fact that homocysteine is an independent risk factor, and has no relationship with any other risk factors.

The editor of the *Journal of the Medical Association of America* (*JAMA*), requests leading medical specialists to comment on the latest most important development in the past year in their particular field. In 1993 Robert M. Russell, MD, of Tufts University, Boston, under the heading Nutrition, placed micronutrients and their role in controlling homocysteine as a factor in heart attacks at the top of his list (*JAMA* 1993; 270: 233-4). This should also have been the cardiologists' theme, but unfortunately was not.

In 1983, Dr Kilmer McCully, the father of this theory, and thereby surely a candidate for the Nobel Prize, published a ninety-page review on homocysteine (*Atherosclerosis Review*, 1983). Another comprehensive review by Ueland and Refsum appeared in the *Journal of Laboratory and Clinical*

Medicine, November 1989. Editorials appeared in *Circulation* (1990; 81: 2004-6) and in *Clinical Chemistry* (1994; 40: 857-8). It is significant to note that *Circulation* is the official journal of the American Heart Association, a body that has jealously guarded against any theory other than the cholesterol-lipid one for atherosclerosis. Undoubtedly this is an admission that the lipid theory cannot explain the total atherosclerosis picture.

Two of the earlier studies need particular attention. In a study of nearly 15 000 American physicians, aged 40 to 84 years, followed up for five years, 271 men who subsequently suffered heart attacks were found to have higher levels of blood homocysteine than a matched control group. Of significance here is that now at least 15 000 American doctors are only too aware of the role of homocysteine in heart attacks (*JAMA* 1992; 268: 877-8).

In a slightly earlier study from Dublin, Ireland, (Clarke R. et al., *NEJM* 1991; 324: 1149-55), four risk factors (high blood homocysteine, high blood cholesterols, high blood pressure and cigarette smoking) were compared in 38 patients with cerebrovascular disease (cerebral thrombosis or haemorrhage, stroke), 25 patients with venous thrombosis or bloodclotting in the legs, and in 60 patients with heart disease (coronary vascular). The two notable results were a 7.7 times higher risk factor for blood homocysteine than blood cholesterol from the heart disease cases, and a 2.3 times higher risk factor for blood homocysteine than high blood pressure for cerebrovascular disease cases (Fig 4.6).

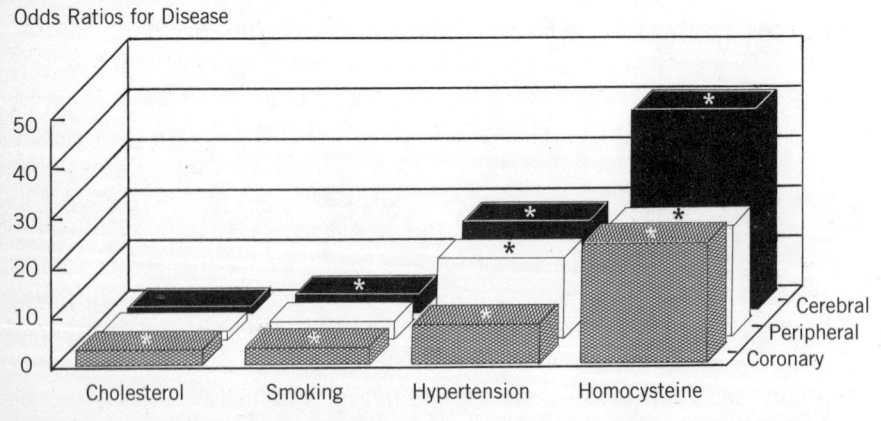

Odds Ratios for Disease

* Indicates statistically significant higher risk

Fig 4.6. Odds ratios for vascular diseases. Comparing the chances of four risk factors – increased cholesterol, smoking, hypertension and increased homocysteine – on three forms of vascular diseases – cerebral (strokes), peripheral (clots in the veins) and coronary (heart attacks). (Clarke et al., *NEJM* 1991; 324: 1149-55.)

One problem in homocysteine research is the method of estimation, the normal blood value being very low, only 1/500th of blood cholesterol. As the differences between normal and abnormal values are small, it was decided to stimulate homocysteine through its precursor, methionine. This increased the difference between the normal and abnormal values considerably, but implies a collection of two blood specimens. One is taken fasting, then methionine at a measured quantity is taken per mouth, and the second blood specimen is drawn after six hours. Now far more reliable results are obtainable, with unfortunately more inconvenience to the patient.

Another important result of high homocysteine blood values is peripheral venous thrombosis or blood clotting in the legs or arms. This is a common modern condition which has increased considerably since food refinement. It usually necessitates antithrombus treatment such as heparin and warfarin, both of which are potentially harmful drugs causing haemorrhage in various parts of the body. Common sense tells us that micronutrients should dissolve and remove the clots through rebalancing prostaglandins, with no danger of haemorrhage.

The First International Congress on Homocysteine, 1995

The homocysteine enthusiasts, now a fast growing group, decided it was time to get together. The First World Congress on Homocysteine was held in Ireland in July, 1995. Delegates came from all over the world to present papers. The largest group was from the USA (33 papers, six from Cleveland, five from Framingham), 23 from the Netherlands, 15 from France, 10 from Norway, seven from Ireland, six from Germany and lesser numbers from Spain, Italy, Australia, Sweden, Switzerland, Denmark, England, Canada, Czechoslovakia, Wales, South Africa, Russia and Poland.

Of the subjects under discussion the largest group concerned the role of the micronutrients. Atherosclerosis, cerebral lesions and venous thrombosis received much attention. Important were the methods of estimation where room for improvement has always been a factor. Accompanying diseases, such as depression, increased and decreased thyroid function, diabetes, chronic fatigue syndrome (Yuppy flu), and spinal tube defects, such as spina bifida, all received attention.

The action mechanism of homocysteine stimulated much interest. How does homocysteine act to increase blood vessel damage, and is this the only mechanism of homocysteine action? This will be discussed later.

An enthusiastic group of researchers, inspired by discussion and co-operation, returned to their respective clinics and laboratories to continue the search for a final answer, not only for coronary heart disease, but also for cerebral and venous thrombosis. It was important that the homocysteine enthusiasts had a precise compact field to work upon, unlike the wide field of cholesterol, lipoproteins, triglycerides, fatty acids and other lipids that the lipidiologists found themselves wading in.

The Statins and Cholesterol: At Last a Lipid Breakthrough

The mid-1990s also brought the first reasonable results in support of the lipid-cholesterol theory by applying drugs that suppressed the formation of cholesterol. These became known as "statins", stat indicating no further formation. Through research by different pharmaceutical laboratories, four types of statins were formed, simvastin, ovastatin, flavastatin and pravastatin. A highly potent regulating enzyme known as **3-hydroxy-3-methyl glutaryl-coenzyme A reductase** is necessary for the formation of cholesterol anywhere in the body. The four statins above all suppress or inhibit this enzyme's function, thereby suppressing the formation of cholesterol.

Cholesterol is, however, no abnormal or toxic substance in the body, but is essential for its numerous functions. In excess, however, it can cause problems. Take the parallel of floods. The latter, caused by water, leads to considerable damage. If we could stop the flow of water from the heavens altogether we could stop floods, but we could also stop the flow to the land, possibly causing more damage through drought than the floods would have done.

In a study over 5.4 years, known as the 4S Study (Scandinavian Simvastin Survival Study) in 4 444 patients who had previously had heart attacks, or suffered from what is known as stabile angina pectoris, 20 to 40 mg of simvastin per day decreased the risk of deaths by 34%, decreased the total cholesterol by 25%, decreased LDL-cholesterol by 35% and increased HDL-cholesterol by 8%. By all standards, these results are quite remarkable. The researchers recommended that the use of simvastin should be restricted to patients with serum cholesterol levels of 5.5 to 8.0 mmol/l (*Lancet* 1994; 344: 1383-89).

A second study known as the West of Scotland Study (*NEJM* 1995; 333: 1301-7) over 4.9 years included 6 595 men aged 45 to 65 years. Pravastatin 40 mg per day was administered. The average results indicated total cholesterol reduced by 20%, LDL-cholesterol reduced by 26%, HDL-cholesterol increased by 5% and triglycerides reduced by 12%. Deaths due to heart attacks were reduced by 28%. Numerous other claims of success were made, such as decreased need for X-rays of the heart vessels (angiography) or for the two surgical procedures on the heart vessels. The treatment with statins would be for life at a conservative cost of £400-600 ($600-900) per year. The researchers advised that the focus should only be on patients with blood cholesterol levels above 6.5 mmol/l.

Great publicity was given to the fact that the doyen of British cardiologists, Prof Michael Oliver, formerly an opponent of the advantage of lowering blood cholesterol, now endorsed the results of the statin studies (*Lancet* 1995; 346: 1378-9). However, in a personal letter to the author he admitted that he had never considered the role of micronutrients in heart disease.

Now for the snags! What about homocysteine, the factor considered to be nearly eight times more of a risk factor than cholesterol? And still more seriously, what about the absolute essential functions of cholesterol?

Cholesterol is an essential element in the wall of every cell in the body, and is required for tissue repair and growth cell turnover. Furthermore, none of the highly important steroid hormones (cholesterol is a steroid) can be formed without the presence of the mother substance, cholesterol. These include all the sex hormones (male testosterone, female oestrogens and progesterones), as well as cortisol which has widespread effects on glucose, on amino acid and fat metabolism, on normal smooth and striated muscle functions and on the formation of blood cells. Cholesterol also forms aldosterone necessary for the control of water balance, and is needed for the manufacture of vitamin D, essential for bone formation. Cortisol and aldosterone are absolutely essential for life (*Lancet* 1991; 388: 666-7). Yet their formations are being prevented by the statins (fig 4.7).

The researchers claim that no adverse effects were noted from the use of statins. Yet they advise that liver function tests should be performed before treatment, every six weeks for the first three months, every eight weeks for the remainder of the first year, and periodically after that every six months.

In any contract one should always read the fine print before accepting. The fine print in the contract between statins and the patient is found in the insert pamphlet in the statin packets. There it states that statins are not to be taken during pregnancy, liver disease or heavy alcohol intake. A large number of other drugs are to be avoided simultaneously, including certain antibiotics and other cholesterol-lowering drugs. They are ineffective in familial hypercholesterolaemia as these patients lack LDL receptors.

The researchers report no adverse effects after 10 years of trials. This is extremely difficult to believe. In the author's experience the majority of cases on 20 to 40 mg per day complain of severe nausea, severe pains and haemorrhages in the muscles and, universal in all, a severe loss of libido. All these

82 • A BLUEPRINT FOR BETTER HEALTH

symptoms are hinted at in the insert pamphlet in the packets. Patients on 10 mg statins per day probably have fewer symptoms, but none of the researchers advise such a low dosage.

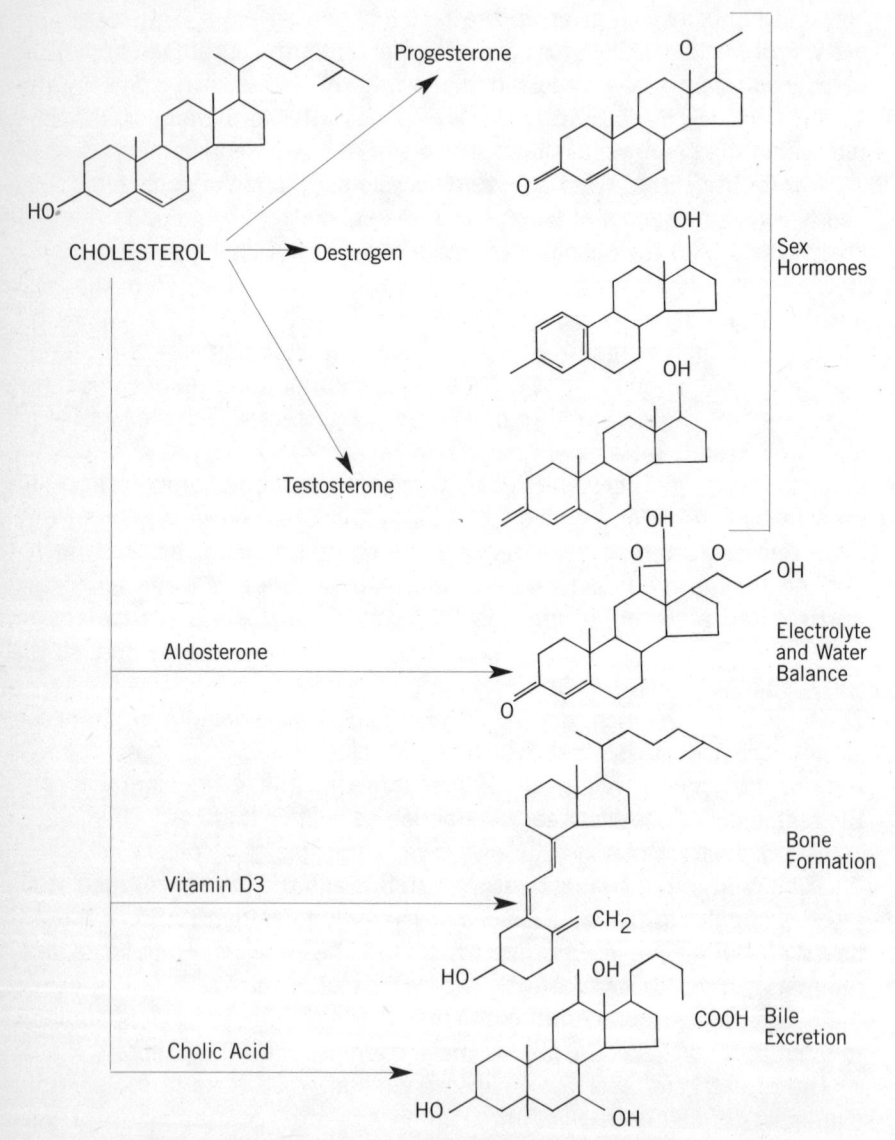

Fig 4.7. Cholesterol and the hormones and structures formed from it. These and their functions will be seriously affected if the formation of the cholesterol molecule is interfered with.

From the viewpoint of adverse effects, did the researchers look at glucose metabolism, at sex functions (sperm counts, menstruation disorders, fertility), water balance (blood electrolytes) and bone function? Naturally one can argue that these symptoms are of lesser importance than deaths from heart attacks. But why administer the above drugs when an alternative is available that has the great potential of being far more effective on cholesterol-lowering, is far less expensive, and has no side effects at all?

In the next chapter the potential of micronutrient therapy will be discussed with the distinct possibility of nearly 100% decrease in heart attacks, normalisation of cholesterol values with no side effects whatsoever, a potential healing of all accompanying metabolic diseases, and, eventually, ideal health at a very reasonable cost.

The Seven Countries Study, 1995 – The Latest

In a follow-up of the Seven Countries Study (*JAMA* 1995; 274: 131-6) a linear relationship, however small, is still noted between coronary heart disease and cholesterol values. However, large differences in "absolute" coronary heart disease deaths at a given cholesterol level indicates that other factors, such as diets typical in cultures with low heart attack risks, are also important. It is therefore suggested that it may be impossible to reduce deaths from heart disease in Northern Europe or elsewhere to levels similar to those in Mediterranean countries by lowering cholesterol alone. This can only be satisfactorily explained by accepting the principle of different basic genetic diets that will not allow foreign genetic races to respond to such new diets.

Table 4.3 illustrates the above principle, taken from the Seven Countries Study.

The above principle is further supported by a study in the Cape Peninsula of South Africa (*SAMJ* 1996; 86: 162) where the total cholesterols of urban Blacks, lately emigrated from the rural areas, have lower total blood cholesterol values (average man 3.98 mmol/l; average woman 4.15 mmol/l) than that of the White, Coloured or Asian population. Furthermore, a study in China (*BMJ* 1995; 311: 409-13) reports that in Shanghai the average blood cholesterol value is 4.2 mmol/l, compared to men in the British Regional Heart Study where average cholesterol values are 6.3 mmol/l.

It is hardly logical to expect all Western communities to lower their

Cohort	Mean Age	Cholesterol mmol/l average	Syst. BP Mean HG	Cigarette Smoking %	Age Standardised 25 Year CHD Mortality Rate
N. Europe	49.4	6.35	144.0	66.8	20.3
USA	49.4	6.20	139.2	59.0	16.0
S. Europe Inland	48.8	5.25	141.3	59.3	9.1
S. Europe Mediterran.	49.4	5.15	137.0	59.2	4.7
Serbia	49.3	4.25	132.5	56.3	7.7
Japan	49.8	4.25	135.0	74.3	3.2

Table 4.3. Follow-up of Seven Countries Study (*JAMA* 1995; 274: 131-6). These results have forced the researchers to modify their original findings, and now accept the fact that cholesterol values are due to cultural differences (in which dietary micronutrients play a leading role).

blood cholesterols to below 5.2 mmol/l, as the lipidiologists have suggested, when we do not know what the average cholesterol values were when heart attacks were rare or even absent, as before 1929.

Other Theories on Atherosclerosis

Prof David Barker of Southhampton has proposed a hypothesis that "a baby's nourishment before birth and during infancy programmes the development of risk factors, such as high blood pressure, fibrinogen concentrations, factor VIII concentrations and glucose intolerance". These are all key considerations in the development of coronary heart disease.

Chlamydia are bacteria which grow only inside cells. Several studies have suggested that antibodies against a strain known as Chlamydia pneumoniae, only described less than ten years ago, is associated with cardiovascular disease (*Circulation* 1993; 87: 1408-9). However, all researchers are careful to state that there is no basis for the conclusion that the bacteria actually causes atherosclerosis.

Both these theories, however, could be incorporated into the theory of micronutrient loss. Babies in modern Western societies start off at gross disadvantages, both from their mother's and their own micronutrient-poor diets. Micronutrients play a decisive role in immunology, giving various bacteria, including chlamydia, a possible role in atherosclerosis via their antibodies.

Gene Therapy for Heart Disease

Geneticists take a futuristic view that sometime all genetic diseases will be curable by replacing abnormal genes with normal genes through germ cell manipulation. Due to the potential danger that such human experiments could get out of hand, only federally approved state clinical trials in the USA and elsewhere are allowed. Profound ethical and philosophical implications are to be considered.

Familial hypercholesterolaemia (FH), the most common dominant condition known, can either be inherited from one parent (heterozygous) or from both (homozygous). In its homozygous form it is usually fatal before the patient is 20 years old. In a genetic experiment liver cells were first isolated from a surgically resected segment of the patient's liver. They were then treated by transferring normal human LDL-receptors to them. The treated cells were then reintroduced into the patient's liver through a catheter originally left in the body at the original resection (*Brit Heart J* 1994; 72: 309-12). In the first patient treated a rapid and sustained reduction in serum LDL and an increase in serum HDL was obtained.

However, since this particular case there has been very little visible advancement in this field.

Geneticists are now suggesting that all genetic factors associated with atherosclerosis, and there are many, should now be researched (*NEJM* 1994; 330: 1129-35). However, the complexity of these genetic disorders is so vast that the cost of treatment to achieve sufficient success would be so excessive as to make it impractical.

With the continuing increase of newly discovered genetic disorders, mainly of a minor or recessive order, it is not unreasonable to believe that the majority of these were suppressed in the presence of sufficient micronutrients controlling the normal metabolism. Should not our first priority be directed at correcting faults which are man-made and which have led to an explosion of Western and modern diseases?

Fat Substitute: Olestra

Olestra, a so-called fat substitute, has now been approved by the US Food and Drug Administration, against the advice of two professors from Harvard and thirty public health specialists. It is a mixture of sugar and vegetable oil, six or seven fatty acids attached to a sucrose molecule. Its use is as a replacement for shortening and cooking oils in the preparation of, amongst other foods, potato chips. Its bulkier shape is too large for intestinal absorption, so it passes through the digestive tract, leaving behind no fat or calories.

The main objection to it is that the fat-soluble vitamins A, D, E and K and caretenoids attach to the Olestra molecule and are swept away along with it. As a condition of its approval, the product must be fortified with the above vitamins (*BMJ* 1996; 312: 270).

A number of objections, however, remain. Dietary cholesterol plays a very minor role in atherosclerosis, only 15% in Western communities responding to a lower dietary cholesterol. The eight-times bigger risk factor, homocysteine, cannot be decreased. Furthermore, the danger of part of the molecule being absorbed brings a new foreign body into play, thereby increasing the danger of cancer. No, there is a far more inexpensive and effective treatment for lowering blood cholesterol, as well as decreasing heart attacks.

The Pharmaceutical Industry: Friend or Foe?

The book, *The Diseases of Civilisation* by Brian Inglis, Hodder and Stoughton, 1981, has the following notable paragraph, p. 264: "It is never easy for any organisation whose members share a set of beliefs and attitudes to recognise that they are becoming irrelevant to the needs of the community. In the case of the medical profession it is made all the more difficult, because it is sustained in many of those beliefs and attitudes by one of the most powerful empires in the world: the pharmaceutical industry. The 'wonder drug' era from the 1930s to the 1950s forged an alliance between the profession and the industry. It has since led to the industry achieving an unprecedented and dangerous measure of control over the profession."

In 1994 Representative Ron Wyden (Democrat, Oregon) requested the General Accounting Office (GAO) to determine whether drug companies' acquisitions of pharmacy benefit management (PBM) companies would drive up the costs. The report said that it had found some dubious practices (*Lancet* 1995; 546: 1416).

The GAO found that the five largest PBMs manage benefits for more than 80% of enrollees in PBM plans. Of these five, three are owned by pharmaceutical companies. These companies naturally would support their own drugs, and all three companies were inclined to this procedure, not necessarily putting forward the least expensive drugs. This is a procedure which is unacceptable, another example of pharmaceutical companies dominating the medical profession.

One company had to pay 1.9 million US dollars to seventeen states in a settlement. It has also been stated that PBMs are helping to drive pharmacists out of business.

It is reported that Swiss drug groups Sandoz and Ciba-Geigy plan to merge in what would be the world's most expensive deal (*BMJ* 1996; 312: 656). Guess who will be the losers.

CHAPTER 5

A COMPLETE THEORY ON ATHEROSCLEROSIS

A good scientific theory should be explicable to a barmaid.
PROF ERNEST RUTHERFORD, SCIENTIST

Putting a Disease into Reverse

Any vehicle entering into a dead-end street has only one sensible way of escape: to reverse. It has little chance of advancement by attempting to force its way amongst the different backyards and fences. The same principle applies to metabolic diseases, including atherosclerosis.

Yet it is precisely through the route of backyards and fences that the majority of researchers have attempted to escape the seeming inevitability of heart attacks. Desperate measures, such as destroying an important fuel, cholesterol, have so many potential and dangerous side effects, that the treatment could be worse than the illness.

In this chapter the author will attempt to convince the reader – as he himself has become convinced through personal clinical evidence – that a simple inexpensive reversal of the atherosclerosis build-up could potentially lead to a near eradication of this disease. It is tragic that totally inadequate studies on many thousands of candidates or volunteers, consuming enormously high costs, have little to show over many decades.

Granted that new facts on lately discovered risk factors have taken a long time to become scientifically accepted, it still remains tragic that most of the older theories are kept alive by persons and practices for whom commercial considerations are uppermost. The final effect is that the patient is the loser, in terms of both health and money.

Time Factors in Western Disease Development

Genetics of man and his predecessors started at the beginning of life some 2 500 million years ago. This included genetics of structures developing according to available foods. These foods underwent corresponding change, itself subject to genetics and climate, leading to a constant change in receptors and metabolic structures in humans and animals.

Some 10 000 years ago, perhaps longer, man came to recognise plants which provide grains, and that by cultivating them he could change his primary hunter's habits to the more tranquil life of gatherer. But if he could gather grains, why not also animals? Soon he came to domesticate certain animals and to derive the benefits of cow milk, fowl eggs, butter and cultivated animal meat. Naturally this diet varied with time, and with it man's genetic metabolic pathways and receptors. This latter process was undeniably thorough, but also painfully slow, taking approximately 1 000 years or 30 to 40 generations to arrive at meaningful change.

The ingredients of successful metabolism have been proved to be an optimum combination of macronutrients and micronutrients, the former being proteins, fats and carbohydrates, and the latter vitamins and minerals. Up to 1880 the macronutrients probably varied far more in various geographical areas than did the micronutrients. However, with the introduction of the roller mill in that year, the picture changed dramatically. Human metabolism now lost on the average over 60% of its absolutely essential micronutrients, the co-factors of its approximately 2 500 enzymes. The body's metabolism, if not coming to a standstill, was at least grossly affected. Diseases that were previously extremely rare or perhaps even absent, developed to become the most common diseases of our time.

As refinement spread to lesser developed areas of the world, its effects became locally apparent, and today we have few regions where refinement has not spread its menacing effect.

An alarming increase in world populations, and with it a dramatic increase in the necessary foods to feed the masses, led to further unfortunate food manufacturing procedures. Food canning came into general use around 1900. Before any food can be canned it has to undergo a heating process, leading to partial destruction of certain vitamins (Gruberg and Raymond, *Beyond Cholesterol Vitamin B6*, Arteriosclerosis and Your Heart, 1981). The wonder of natural refrigeration has been present since the ice age, but that of general household refrigeration only since World War II, 1939-45. This, too, has led to vitamin losses. Add to this the effects of additives, plus the replacement of organic fertilisation by artificial means, and the stage has been set where all micronutrients, all present at optimum values before 1880, have been lost at values of over 60% to over 90% in individual cases.

The Role of Genetics

It is important to repeat the role of genetics in diet. Remember the thirteen genetic races which developed according to climate and foods available locally in different geographical regions of the world.

The important factors here are the receptor systems which have adapted to receive and further the metabolism of a variation of foods or chemical structures developing from them. Remember also the time-factor of 1 000 years or 30 to 40 generations required for these genetic factors to become predominant in a race. Genetic factors are hardly ever 100% dominant in a genetic race. Lesser figures of, for example, perhaps 80%, could be present for a specific dominant gene, allowing some genes not to conform to that of the majority, as was seen in the lactase and alcohol dehydrogenase enzymes.

It is estimated that approximately 30% of all human genes are heterozygous, i.e. these genes differ in their structure in different persons. All the other genes are identical in all persons.

Examples of dietary problems which can be clarified on the basis of genetics are the differences in response to alcohol intake, whether fresh or fermented milk should be used, why butter is acceptable and not margarine, why full-cream milk is acceptable and not 2% cream-milk, why eggs do not increase blood cholesterols, and why cholesterol-containing foods do not increase blood cholesterols in races that have had a high cholesterol intake for thousands of years.

The Role of Micronutrients

It is important to repeat that micronutrients are essential for the normal function of probably every enzyme in the body. With losses of 60% to over 90% of micronutrients through modern food processing and allied procedures, little doubt exists that this enforced slowing down of every metabolic pathway in the body must inevitably lead to metabolic diseases. Two metabolic pathways are particularly important.

The **methionine-homocysteine pathway** is primarily developed to provide methyl molecules and to develop an essential muscle and tissue protein, cysteine, whose function is to strengthen the body's ligaments and connective tissue. However, due to a shortage of micronutrients, specifically vitamin B6, vitamin B12, folic acid and magnesium, homocysteine increases in the blood, and thereby aids in inititiating atherosclerosis and furthering thrombosis.

The second metabolic pathway affected has far wider effects, in so far as it controls the whole delicate **essential fatty acid-prostaglandin-thromboxane-leukotriene** balanced metabolism, the eics. The all-important enzyme here is delta-6-desaturase, stimulating the reaction linoleic acid to gamma-linolenic acid (GLA). Five micronutrients are essential here, vitamin B6, vitamin C, magnesium, zinc and nicotinic acid.

The importance of the above-mentioned micronutrients can be summarised as follows:

> Total number of enzymes approximately 2 500;
> At least 420 require nicotinic acid;
> At least 300 require magnesium;
> At least 200 require zinc;
> At least 120 require vitamin B6.

Of other micronutrients the figures are as follows:
> At least 400 require phosphate;
> At least 120 require vitamin B2 (riboflavine);
> At least 60 require iron;
> At least 25 require sulphur;
> At least 18 require manganese;
> At least 18 require copper;
> At least 10 require vitamin B1 (thiamine).
> At least 10 require calcium.

(*International Congress on Enzymes*, IUB 1984, Webb E.C.)

Antioxidant Effect of Micronutrients

Although life could not have developed without oxygen, an overdose (as with any other substance) can also be harmful. If a person receives pure oxygen in a closed circuit for too long, as with a too-tight oxygen mask in a hospital, it could be fatal. Many tissues in the body, such as blood vessel walls, stomach linings, certain proteins, red blood cell membranes and many more, can all be harmed by chemical compounds with a too-high oxygen content, as for example, oxidised cholesterol. But man, in order to survive, has been programmed with built-in antioxidants, the life-saving vitamins C, E and A, and the latter's precursor, beta-carotene.

At the International Congress on Antioxidant Vitamins and Beta-Carotene held in London, 2-4 October 1989, various conditions associated with a shortage of antioxidants were discussed. They included heart disease, stom-

92 • A BLUEPRINT FOR BETTER HEALTH

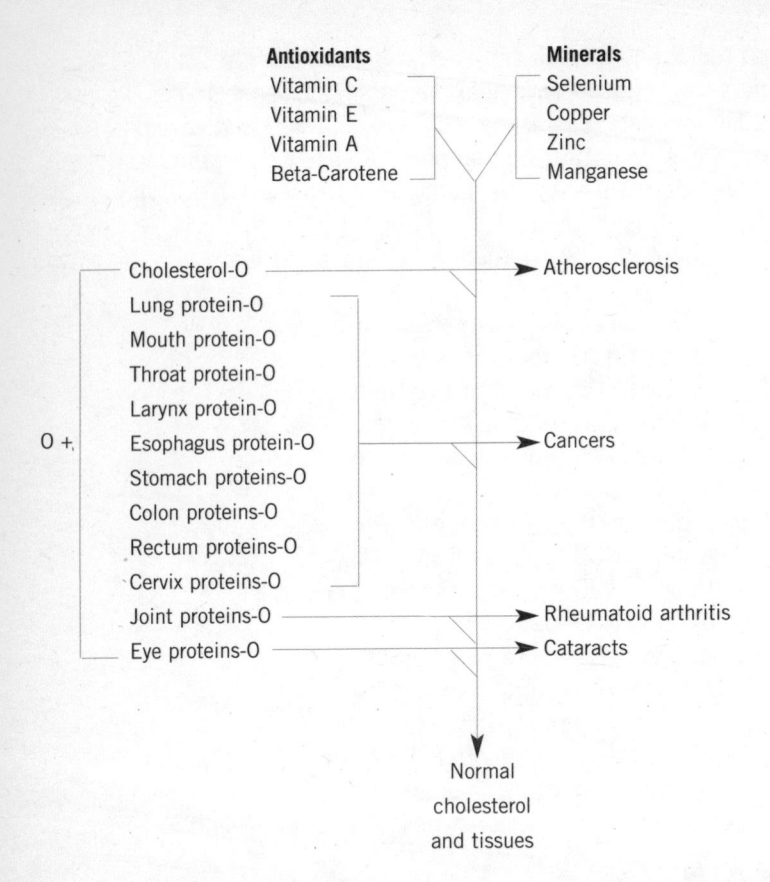

```
                Antioxidants        Minerals
                Vitamin C           Selenium
                Vitamin E           Copper
                Vitamin A           Zinc
                Beta-Carotene       Manganese
```

```
        ┌─ Cholesterol-O ─────────────► Atherosclerosis
        │  Lung protein-O
        │  Mouth protein-O
        │  Throat protein-O
        │  Larynx protein-O
 O +  ──┤  Esophagus protein-O ──────► Cancers
        │  Stomach proteins-O
        │  Colon proteins-O
        │  Rectum proteins-O
        │  Cervix proteins-O
        │  Joint proteins-O ──────────► Rheumatoid arthritis
        └─ Eye proteins-O ────────────► Cataracts

                        ▼
                     Normal
                   cholesterol
                   and tissues
```

Fig 5.1. The protective effects of antioxidants and minerals in preventing atherosclerosis, cancers, rheumatoid arthritis and cataracts.

ach cancer, eye cataracts, rheumatoid arthritis, Parkinson's disease, loss of immunity, ageing, melanomas (skin pigment cancer), and certain other cancers, including lung cancer (Fig 5.1).

It is important to realise that antioxidant vitamins are all solely oil-soluble vitamins, i.e. they are only soluble in oil and not in water. Unwittingly oils have been removed from many foods in order to "lengthen the shelf life" of such foods. This is particularly important in the most commonly eaten grain, wheat. "Whole-wheat bread" is indeed a misnomer, for 3% of its total has been removed, the vital 3% containing the oil-soluble antioxidant vitamins. This loss can be remedied by adding whole wheatgerm daily to the diet.

Antioxidant research has a high international priority at present, but it must be emphasised that antioxidants are in fact nothing else but micronutrients.

Four minerals are also known to have antioxidant functions; selenium, copper, zinc and manganese. Much interest is presently concentrated upon the effects of individual antioxidants with some controversial effects. Common sense tells us that the antioxidants should be seen as factors acting in unison with many other micronutrients.

The Role of Homocysteine

This has already been fully discussed. It should be emphasised that it is a risk factor entirely independent of lipid risk factors. Furthermore it is approximately eight times more important than blood cholesterol in contributing to coronary heart disease, and of 2.3 times more significance than high blood pressure for cerebral vascular disease or strokes.

Homocysteine's role in deep venous thrombosis or "clots in the legs" has only recently been recognised as a critical factor in this deadly vascular disease, which has been on the increase in industrial populations. Previous accusations levelled at tight clothing have been proven inconclusive.

The homocysteine theory is still bugged by certain problems. The pathological mechanism is still not clear. In the more severe but rare congenital homocystinuria, the main factor is probably endothelial damage, i.e. damage to the inner layers of the blood vessels. In the noncongenital homocysteine increase in blood, hyperhomocysteinaemia, as seen in ordinary atherosclerosis and heart attacks, the mechanism causing atherosclerosis is still uncertain.

Theories suggest a wide number of possible effects. One fairly widely accepted view is that because of its sulphur-containing structure or composition, homocysteine acts as an oxidant. Besides having a toxic effect on tissues, it also causes a toxic cholesterol to form, thereby damaging blood vessel walls.

Blood clotting is a complicated procedure in which numerous factors, possibly as many as fifteen to twenty, play a role. Homocysteine appears to reduce the binding of certain blood-clotting factors to the blood vessel wall, thus allowing blood to clot more readily, which is undesirable.

It would also appear that certain enzymes in blood vessel walls are inhibited by a high blood homocysteine. This leads to an increase of elastic and collagen tissues in the walls, incorrectly folded proteins in the walls, and decreased breakdown of homocysteine itself, leading to a veritable vicious circle of increased homocysteine (Fig 5.2).

94 • A BLUEPRINT FOR BETTER HEALTH

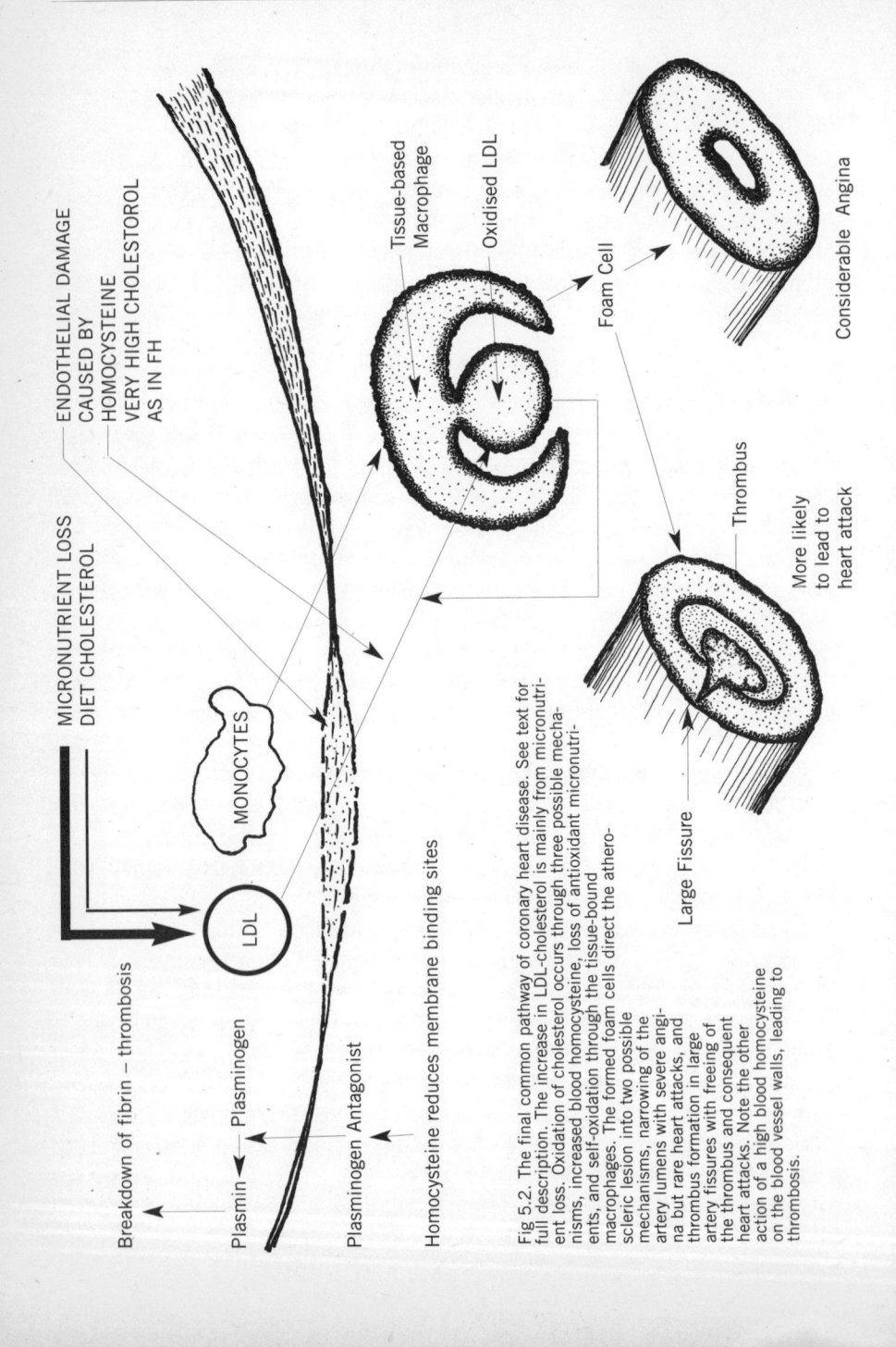

Fig 5.2. The final common pathway of coronary heart disease. See text for full description. The increase in LDL-cholesterol is mainly from micronutrient loss. Oxidation of cholesterol occurs through three possible mechanisms, increased blood homocysteine, loss of antioxidant micronutrients, and self-oxidation through the tissue-bound macrophages. The formed foam cells direct the atherosclerotic lesion into two possible mechanisms, narrowing of the artery lumens with severe angina but rare heart attacks, and thrombus formation in large artery fissures with freeing of the thrombus and consequent heart attacks. Note the other action of a high blood homocysteine on the blood vessel walls, leading to thrombosis.

All the above mechanisms are described in the summary of the International Conference on Homocysteine Metabolism, 1995, reported in the *Irish Journal of Medical Science* 1995; I64: Supplement 15.

The Cause of High Blood Total and LDL-Cholesterol

Lipid researchers have stubbornly persisted in attributing a high blood cholesterol to a high dietary cholesterol. Despite the apparent logic of this assumption, study after study in Western communities has, without exception, proved this to be largely incorrect. Only one out of seven persons of Western populations have responded in any way by increasing their blood cholesterols. Genetics over thousands of years have obviously developed a defence mechanism, either in gut absorption or in liver metabolism or in both, to counter increased dietary cholesterol.

Yet it is a well-known fact that communities on a Westernised diet, which includes a high cholesterol intake, have increased their average blood cholesterols to levels well above those of African, Indo-Dravidian and Sino-Japanese races. What is the explanation if dietary cholesterol is not to blame?

The emphasis on total cholesterol, LDL and HDL-cholesterol, has led to a neglect of another most important subdivision of cholesterol, **free cholesterol** and **conjugated or esterified cholesterol.** This division is based partly on solubility, esterified cholesterol being far less soluble than free cholesterol. Consequently esterified cholesterol is situated to the centre of both LDL and HDL-lipoprotein molecules. The more soluble free cholesterol, situated peripherally, can therefore appear free in the blood, and is consequently able to be excreted in the bile.

An ester indicates any substance combined with a fatty acid. Unsaturated fatty acids are readily metabolised further, for which micronutrients are necessary. Saturated fatty acids are not easily metabolised further as they act as end products.

In esterified cholesterol, always comprising two-thirds of the total, at least 12 fatty acids are present. The strict laws of chemical balance keep this ratio of conjugated to free cholesterol constant. If the one increases or decreases the other must likewise change. The most important of these fatty acids is an old friend, linoleic acid, the most common polyunsaturated fatty acid in the human body, and the same one upon which the all-important enzyme, delta-6-desaturase, acts to initiate the just-as-important prostaglandin 1 pathway. The micronutrients needed are the same: vitamin B6, vitamin C, zinc, magnesium and nicotinic acid.

NAME	FATTY ACIDS SHORTHAND FORMULA	% (1)	% (2)
Myristic	14:0	1.04	1.04
Palmitic	16:0	12.74	10.64
Palmitoleic*	16:1	4.57	4.04
Stearic	18:0	1.51	0.93
Oleic*	18:1	21.27	19.66
Linoleic*	18:2w-6	49.17	53.06
Gamma-Linolenic*	18:3w-6	0.86	0.95
Alpha-Linolenic*	18:3w-3	0.83	1.09
Dihomogammalinoleic*	20:3w-6	0.61	0.66
Arachidonic*	20:4w-6	4.97	5.52
Eicosapentaenoic*	20:5w-3	1.64	0.96
Docosahexanoic*	22:6w-3	0.80	0.56

* Indicates fatty acids which can be further metabolised by micronutrients.

Table 5.1. Average percentages of fatty acids in cholesterol esters from two references (*Am J Clin Nutr* 1994; 59: 364-70; *Am J Clin Nutr* 1984; 42: 708-13).

Table 5.1 lists the fatty acids and their percentages from two references. Only approximately 15% of the fatty acids cannot be metabolised due to their full saturation. The other 85% can all be metabolised, most certainly requiring diverse micronutrients for their actions. A simple mathematical sum indicates 85% of 66% = 56% of the total cholesterol is under biochemical control of micronutrients.

Granted that at present the micronutrients for the majority of the above fatty acids are unknown, little doubt exists that they are necessary, and will in time be discovered.

Now it becomes clear that with a micronutrient shortage, including the five mentioned micronutrients, linoleic acid and the other unsaturated fatty acids combined to cholesterol cannot be metabolised adequately. The result is a rise in esterified cholesterol and a simultaneous rise in free cholesterol due to the laws of chemical balance. Thus the total cholesterol increases.

Should sufficient micronutrients be present, all the unsaturated fatty acids can be metabolised adequately, leading to a decrease in esterified, free and total cholesterol. This condition was undoubtedly present before the introduction of food refining, explaining the lower cholesterol, LDL, HDL and total in primitive undeveloped races.

Considering the above facts, a strong case can be made out for the loss of micronutrients as the most important cause of a rise in blood cholesterol.

Experimental Proof

The first recorded experiment on humans that micronutrients could lower blood cholesterol was that of Brusis (*Fortschr Med*, 1985) when he administered Sudalipid, a tablet containing a magnesium-vitamin B6-gluconate, 150 mg per day, to four groups of patients with high blood fats. Three of these groups had genetic conditions, one being familial hypercholesterolaemia (FH), the most common genetic disease recorded. The fourth group was considered high-risk due to high blood fats without known genetic conditions (Table 5.2).

	FH		Type II B		Type IV		High Risk	
Cases	45		142		19		45	
	Chol	Tgl	Chol	Tgl	Chol	Tgl	Chol	Tgl
Basic	9.6	1.39	9.9	3.44	5.8	5.80	7.2	4.54
After 4 weeks	8.3	1.38	8.2	2.75	5.5	4.35	6.5	3.42
After 8 weeks	7.3	1.24	7.4	2.49	5.2	3.31	6.1	2.78

(All values in mmol/l)

Table 5.2. The effect of magnesium-vitamin B6-glutamate (Sudalipid), 150 mg per day on four groups with high blood lipids. The first three are of genetic conditions, including familial hypercholesterolaemia, and the fourth the common high-risk atherosclerosis. Note that the lipids are not lowered to levels below normal as the effect is only on the esterified cholesterol (Brusis, *Fortschr Med*, 1985).

All responded remarkably well over a period of eight weeks, showing decreases in the high-risk group of 15% cholesterol, and in the FH group of 23%. Unfortunately no control group on placebos was included. Lipid researchers were quick to invalidate the results due to the absence of the control group. Nevertheless, the results are remarkable when compared to dietary and other drug attempts at lowering the cholesterol.

Previous reference has been made to the often stated "saturated fats increase the cholesterol, especially when replacing carbohydrates". Here again, this clearly points to a decrease of micronutrients, which are in their highest concentration in complex carbohydrates, as the factor responsible for the rise in blood cholesterol, not the saturated fats.

This has now been confirmed by Ascherio and co-workers of Boston Medical School, who indicate clearly that an increase in saturated fats does not increase the cholesterol (*BMJ* 1996; 313: 84-90).

The original Seven Countries Study had suggested that it was the animal fats that increased deaths from heart attacks, while vegetable fats lowered deaths, and included USA statistics. In 1978 Dr Mary Enig and colleagues reported that during the time that heart attack deaths increased in the USA, a decrease in the per capita intake of saturated and animal fats took place, with an increase in per capita intake of unsaturated and vegetable fats (*Fed Proceedings* 1978; 37: 2215-20). This once more invalidates the original conclusions of the Seven Countries Study. Fig 5.3 A and B indicate Dr Enig's findings, facts which support the role of micronutrient loss as a causative factor in heart disease. Note the period of 40 years between the time that micronutrient loss reached its maximum in 1890, and the initial rise in deaths from heart attacks in 1929.

Personal Experience of the Author

Since 1982 the author and colleagues have conducted research on the effects of micronutrients on heart disease, with expanding interests in other metabolic diseases. Advice to certain colleagues on the use of micronutrients led to a serendipitous discovery that an inexpensive multimicronutrient supplementation led to a dramatic decrease in blood cholesterol. The mechanism has been explained previously.

Four patients on different occasions consulted the author after they had been told that immediate bypass operations on their coronary arteries were necessary. The author prescribed an inexpensive multimicronutrient tablet once daily. However, as nearly all of these multimicronutrient tablets contained insufficient magnesium, according to the Recommended Daily Average (RDA), this mineral was added at a dosage of approximately 150 mg per day.

Within weeks the symptoms of angina in all four patients had disappeared, and no heart surgery was necessary. In one case, a doctor's wife, an X-ray of the patient's coronary arteries (angiogram) after one year's treatment revealed a remarkable improvement in the blood flow through the arteries, "the best improvement he had ever seen" according to the patient's cardiologist.

A double blind study on patients with high cholesterols (above 6.7 mmol/l) carried out on free-living persons in the northern suburbs of Cape Town and Hermanus, South Africa, revealed a 6.8% average decrease in total cholesterol in 35 persons within six weeks as compared to a 2.2% decrease in 39 persons in a placebo group. Many participants volunteered information

A COMPLETE THEORY ON ATHEROSCLEROSIS • 99

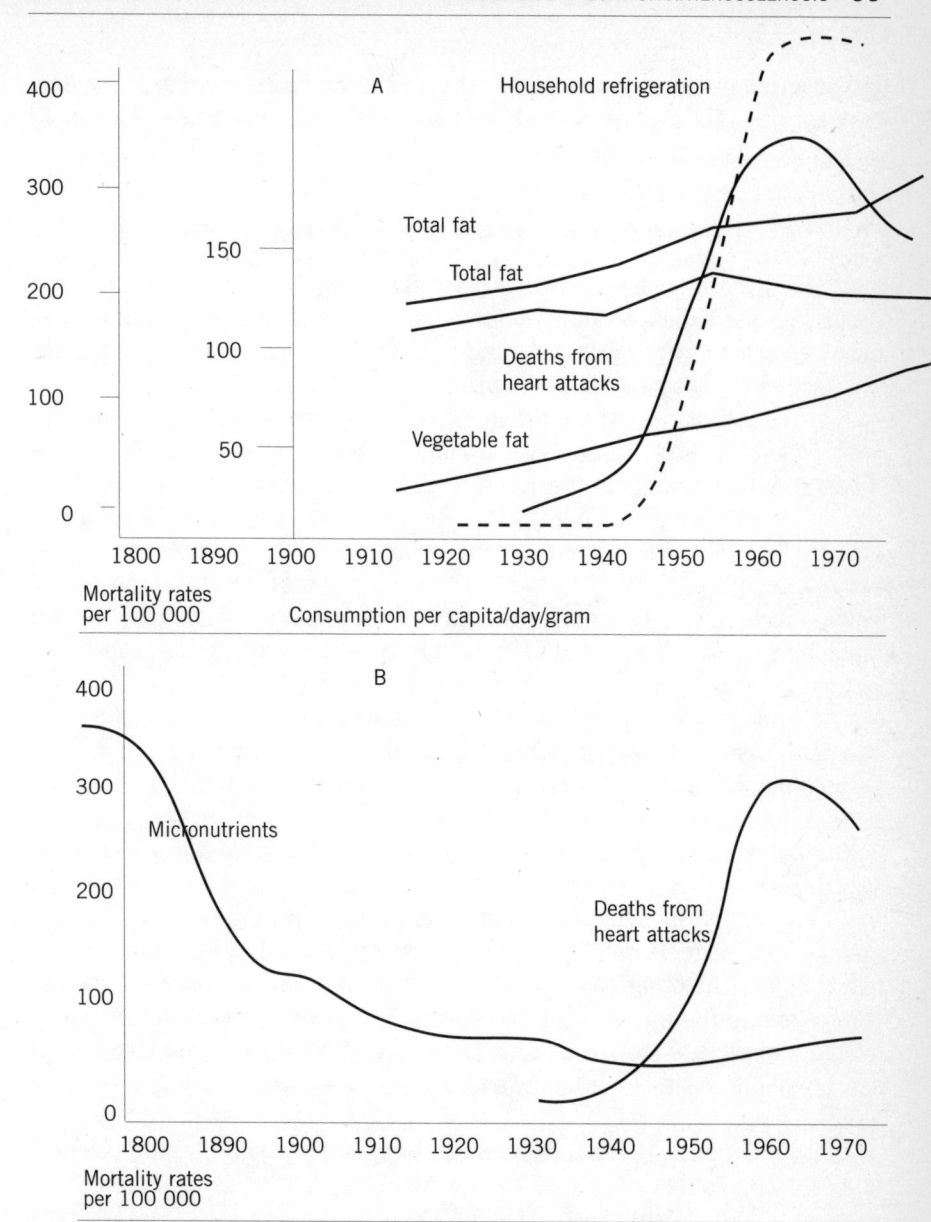

Fig 5.3 A. A comparison of the death rates from heart attacks (unbroken line) compared to the time of roller mills' introduction (1880), general canning introduction (1900), household refrigeration (broken line) and the consumption per capita of total fat, animal fat and vegetable fat, all figures from the USA (M. Enig, 1978).
B. Comparing nutrient loss (theoretically derived) with heart attack deaths. Note the 40-year interval between the commencement of each.

on the improvement of symptoms in other metabolic diseases, such as rheumatoid arthritis and hypertension. Many remarked also on a sense of renewed energy that they had experienced.

The Final Common Pathway of Coronary Heart Disease

Ever since the increase in deaths from heart attacks in 1929 the medical profession has expended much effort in attempting to solve the problem. In 1981 an article by P.N. Hopkins and R.R. Williams featured 246 suggested risk factors for heart disease (*Atherosclerosis* 1981; 40: 1-52).

Fig 5.2 summarises the most modern conception of the development of atherosclerosis. Prof Eugene Braunwald, Professor of Medicine at Harvard Medical School, explains the role of lipids as follows: The atherosclerotic lesions develop as a consequence of the movement of monocyte cells and LDL-cholesterol through pores or small openings in the damaged inner layers of blood vessels. The monocyte now becomes a tissue-bound macrophage. LDL-cholesterol now undergoes oxidation and acts on the macrophage. The latter now ingests the cholesterol molecule, eventually forming what is known as a foam cell.

The oxidation of LDL-cholesterol is probably via homocysteine, as well as due to a loss of antioxidant micronutriets, vitamin D, vitamin E, vitamin A, beta-carotene, selenium, copper, zinc and magnesium. Probably this oxidised LDL also causes damage to the endothelial cells.

Current opinion is that coronary heart disease should be divided into two separate conditions. One is the progressive constriction of the artery wall and narrowing of the lumen or opening. When this narrowing reaches approximately 85% of the total, considerable angina can occur, but very rarely a heart attack. The other condition is the eventual development of a large fissure or tear in the thickening arterial wall. This leads to the development of a large thrombus or clot. The latter can either be dissolved spontaneously, or can break off and block a narrowed coronary artery, thus leading to a heart attack.

In the meantime, thrombi or clots can form in the blood. Plasmin is a protein that breaks down fibrin to form a thrombus, but is itself formed from another protein, plasminogen. The clotting of blood is an extremely intricate process, some 12 to 15 structures all playing a role. In the wall of the blood vessel a plasminogen antagonist is present, preventing thrombosis. Homocysteine is believed to reduce the membrane binding sites of the plasminogen antagonist, thus favouring the formation of blood clotting.

The Major Mechanisms of Atherosclerosis

The following six mechanisms are of importance here (Fig 5.4):
1. The homocysteine mechanism. This is probably the most important factor leading to damage to the inner layers of the blood vessels (endothelium), to oxidation of LDL-cholesterol and to interference with the normal clotting of blood.
2. The oxidant action, particularly affecting LDL-cholesterol, due to the loss of antioxidants in food manufacturing.

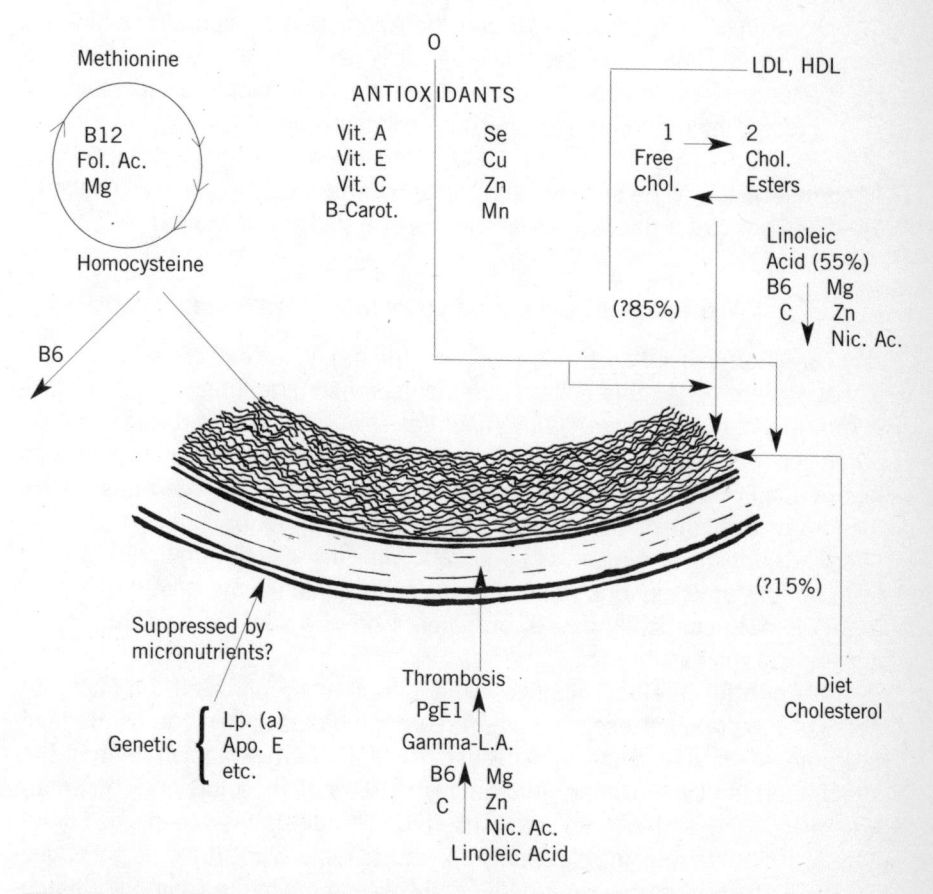

Fig 5.4. The six major mechanisms in the development atherosclerosis. Note that five of the six are due to micronutrient loss.

3. The increase of LDL-cholesterol due to the decrease of micronutrients metabolising the unsaturated fatty acids in cholesterol esters.
4. The increase in dietary cholesterol which in industrialised or Western nations will only affect 1 out of 7 persons. A higher percentage of persons may be affected in primitive races, or in those that have not had a genetic high cholesterol intake.
5. The decrease of dietary micronutrients aiding in the metabolism of linoleic acid leads to a decrease in prostaglandins E1, thereby aggravating the thrombotic process in atherosclerosis.
6. Besides important genetic factors, such as in FH, lesser genetic factors such as lipoprotein (a) and the Apoprotein Es can also play roles in certain heart diseases. However, it is reasonable to believe that the effects of these lesser important genetic factors may be largely suppressed by optimum micronutrient concentrations.

In summary it is to be stressed that of the above six major factors concerning atherosclerosis, five are under the direct influence of micronutrients.

The Treatment and Control of Coronary Heart Disease

Any condition caused by the loss of something, should be able to be cured, if that something is replenished. Common coronary artery disease falls wholly into this category. Little doubt should exist in the mind of the reader that atherosclerotic heart disease can be cured by replacing the micronutrients lost in such large measures. This can occur through two procedures – by a diet with a high micronutrient content, and by supplementation with micronutrients. The diet must be genetic, i.e. it must be applicable to the specific forefather genetic races. However, the replenishment with micronutrients is not genetically based, but should be of a specific amount replacing the lost micronutrients.

It is doubtful whether any diet would sufficiently replace all the micronutients of the prefoodprocessing era. A reasonable calculation can be made of the amount of micronutrients needed for sufficient replenishment if the Recommended Daily Dietary Allowances (RDDA) of the individual micronutrients for men and women are consulted. These RDDAs are revised from time to time but remain reasonably constant (Table 5.3). It would be advisable to partake of all micronutrients daily, in perhaps more than one dosage per day, rather than the individual micronutrients separately. The tablets must not be too large to swallow, or too small to be effective.

In the circumstances of a long absence of dietary micronutrients in certain persons, perhaps that of a lifetime, it would be initially advisable to double up on the dosage for a maximum period of two months, analogous to "priming the body".

Calcium and phosphate are not necessary to be taken in tablet form, as any reasonable diet will contain enough of these minerals in foodstuffs such as milk and vegetables. However, magnesium which has at least 300 co-factor functions in the body needs to be administered in high concentrations, such as an additional 150 mg per day.

Biochemical measurements of micronutrients in the blood, similar to blood cholesterol estimations, are not advised. Such values are inaccurate and do not portray concentrations in the organs and tissues, such as we would wish to know. As an example, organ or tissue magnesium concentrations are only reflected in white blood cells, an estimation for which approximately 50 milliliters of unclotted blood is needed in a highly specialised laboratory. A normal blood magnesium is no reflection of the same in the body tissues. Accept gracefully that you have a micronutrient shortage and take your supplements.

The high micronutrient diet will be discussed in a separate chapter.

	Vit. A ug RE	Vit. D ug	Vit. E mg	Vit. C mg	Thiamine mg	Riboflavin mg	Niacin mg	Vit. B6 mg
Males 25-50 y	1000	5	10	60	1.2	1.4	15	2.0

	Folate ug	Vit. B12 ug	Ca mg	P mg	Mg mg	Fe mg	Zn mg	I ug	Selenium ug
Males 25-50 y	200	200	800	800	350	10	15	150	70

	Copper mg	Manganese mg
Males Adult	1.5-3.0	2.0-5.0

Table 5.3. Recommended daily allowances (1989). Food and Nutrition Board, National Research Council, USA. Women and children differ proportionately, being slightly lower than the figures given here.

Additional Advantages of Micronutrients

Little doubt exists that other metabolic diseases have also increased phenomenally since the advent of roller mills, canning and household refrigeration. These include high blood pressure, venous thrombosis, diabetes mellitus type II, rheumatoid arthritis, cancer, allergies, osteoporosis, obesity, diverticulitis, spastic colon, depression, dental caries and others. The loss of micronutrients has a profound effect on the prostaglandin metabolism and its inbalance, especially if it is chronic, leading to all of the above-mentioned metabolic diseases.

It is of importance to note that the treatment of hypertension by the conventional drugs does not lessen heart attacks. Therapy with micronutrients should lower the incidence of both heart attacks and hypertension.

Frequently, persons in their sixties present individually with coronary heart disease, expressed by angina, high blood pressure, diabetes mellitus type II, rheumatoid arthritis, osteoporosis, cancer and allergies, all present in one individual. We pity such an individual for his or her many simultaneous illnesses, but the logical cause of each is one and the same, a micronutrient shortage. The author has seen many of these cases who are either cured or considerably improved in all their illnesses with simple and inexpensive micronutrient therapy, and a genetic micronutrient diet.

Folic acid supplementation. The USA Department of Health and Human Services and the Food and Drug Administration will require folic acid to be added to all enriched foods from 1 January 1998. All women of child-bearing age should eat at least 400 ug folic acid daily to reduce their risk of giving birth to children with neural tube defects (spina bifida). Folic acid will be added to most enriched breads, flours, corn meals, pastas, rice and other grain products. Folic acid has been proved to be the most effective micronutrient to lower blood homocysteine. Consequently we can expect a dramatic drop in heart attacks. Let us take care that the lipidiologists do not attribute this to statins. Furthermore it can be expected that a 25-50% reduction in risk of orofacial clefts (lips and palates) will occur, as proven at the Children's Hospital in Oakland (*Lancet* 1995; 345: 393-6).

CHAPTER 6

LIFESTYLE

The unfortunate thing about this world is that good habits are so much easier to give up than bad habits.
SOMERSET MAUGHAN

Introduction

Without lessening the primary importance of micronutrients in warding off modern diseases, it would be so much less complicated if the battle against ill health excluded an incorrect lifestyle. Little doubt exists that a healthy mind fosters a healthy body. You can follow the healthiest possible diet but it will be of little avail if it has to battle against the physical, moral and mental afflictions brought on by human weaknesses.

Under aspects of a negative lifestyle we have to include smoking and the misuse of alcohol, while a positive lifestyle embraces an active mind and useful hands, giving satisfaction physically and mentally to the individual and his fellow beings.

A number of lifestyle trials have been initiated by different study groups, and their reported results have been highly enlightening ("The Lifestyle Heart Trial", *Lancet*, 21 July 1990). Old age is no hindrance to a healthy lifestyle, and people in their seventies frequently derive the most benefit.

For medical purposes, lifestyle encompasses mainly four aspects of life; smoking, alcohol, exercise and relaxation. Though frequently the butt of jokes, the numerous personal tragedies of individuals afflicted by negative lifestyle are to be likened to a life sometimes worse than death.

Smoking

Little if anything can be said in favour of cigarette smoking. "It gives you poise", but a pen in the hand gives you much more. "It is so sophisticated", if you are willing to massacre definitions. "It does so much for you", yes, if you only knew what. "It is so macho and makes such a man of you", yes, son, and a very old man at the prime of your life.

Cigarette smoking is undoubtedly closely associated with lung cancer: 1% of Westerners develop it after smoking 20 cigarettes per day for 20 years. Persons who smoke 60 cigarettes per day for 40 years have a 20% chance of developing lung cancer (Branch W.T., *Office Practice of Medicine*, 1987). This does not mean that the other 80% are not affected by smoking. They are candidates for emphysema (four times more common than in nonsmokers), chronic bronchitis and coronary heart disease. Cigar and pipe smokers may be less prone to lung disease, but they have increased danger of mouth cancer. Evidence is now accumulating that smoking is not the only factor in lung cancer, but that a refined diet may play an additional role (Davis D.L., *Lancet*, 25 Aug 1990).

The death rate from coronary heart disease is 70% higher in smokers than in nonsmokers (Branch W.T., 1987). Fortunately, after ten years of abstinence from smoking, the death rate from heart attacks returns to the same figures as for those who never smoked. Evidence clearly associates cigarette smoking with duodenal ulcers. These ulcers will not heal while smoking continues, and it is useless to treat ulcers while the patient continues smoking. Cigarette smoking also leads to hoarseness, sleeplessness and intermittent narrowing of the arteries of the arms and legs, a condition known as intermittent claudication. This could lead to gangrene and amputation of the legs. Furthermore, the effect on oral contraceptive pill users is that smoking increases the excess annual deaths three- to sevenfold (American College of Science and Health, 1990).

How does smoking affect the heart? A special report (*Arterioscler.* 1985; 5: 678A-82A, Grady et al.) states that it probably damages the artery wall, allowing more cholesterol to be deposited. It also reduces HDL-cholesterol, causes disturbances in the heart rhythm and increases the likelihood of developing atherosclerosis in the abdominal aorta and arteries of the legs.

Compared to nonsmokers, men who smoked 25 or more cigarettes per day had a relative increased risk of 1.45 in prostate cancer (*Am J Epid* 1996; 143: 1002-5).

Ex-smokers and relatives of smokers are now turning to legislative action in claiming against tobacco companies. In Britain lawyers have taken up claims for 200 people with illnesses linked to tobacco. Legal aid was granted to a man who lost a leg due to Buerger's disease, a condition aggravated by smoking. Further aid has been granted to other individual cases.

In the USA two massive actions were initiated in which several states were suing tobacco companies for the cost of caring for patients. Fifty law firms banded together to bring an action on behalf of all smokers. The cases are not based on a failure to warn, but mainly on failure to minimise risks by not reducing the tar and nicotine content of cigarettes, when they knew the danger at least 30 years ago. (*BMJ* 1995; 310: 550). This case was defeated in the US law courts on grounds of being too broad a charge. However, the anti-smoking associations are regrouping to renew their legal attack on the tobacco industries.

To stop smoking calls for a lot of effort. The following suggestions could help.
1. Don't carry cigarettes on you; buy a limited number; put them out after a few inhalations.
2. Try to stop for one day at a time.
3. Don't empty dirty ashtrays. This will create an unpleasant association with smoking.
4. Substitute some form of exercise for smoking.
5. Avoid alcohol, which relaxes your determination not to smoke.
6. Induce a friend to stop at the same time.
7. Smoke excessively for one or two days to create an unpleasant association with cigarettes, and then stop abruptly.
8. Let your doctor or an acquaintance take you to an emphysema ward in a hospital to view the irreversible suffering of those desperate patients.
9. If all else fails, ask to see "a smoker's lung" in a postmortem pathology laboratory. That will shock you.

The rule should therefore be No Smoking.

Alcohol

The debate on alcohol use has hotted up considerably within the last few years, especially in its role as a possible factor preventing heart attacks. The American College of Science and Health recommended in 1990 that if alcohol is used, it should be used responsibly and in moderation. The definitions of the latter are controversial. Between 12 and 14% of regular drinkers become problem drinkers, and at least 5% become alcoholics. In genetic races not programmed for alcohol (Blacks, American Indians, Orientals) these percentages are higher.

The major problem with alcohol lies in establishing the boundary between too much and enough, especially with differing genetic races. The exhilaration of climbing Mount Everest could end in disaster if you have not taken enough precautions against falling over the top.

Research indicates that up to a maximum of 45 g of alcohol per day is efficiently used by the liver for body metabolism. More than that is toxic to the body. In 1987 the Royal Medical Colleges of London set safe limits for alcohol intake at 21 units per week for men and 14 units per week for women. (1 Unit = 12 g alcohol = half-pint beer = 1 glass of wine; *BMJ* 1996; 312: 7-9). Alcohol increases HDL, lowers plasma fibrinogen and reduces platelet activity, all advantageous to the heart.

Towards the end of 1994 the World Health Organisation (WHO) came out with a strong criticism of the concept that alcohol should be considered a preventative factor against heart attacks. "We are seeking to demystify advertising that says alcohol is good for your health, and to debunk the idea that to have a drink per day will keep the doctor away. There is no minimum threshold below which alcohol can be consumed without any risk. Alcohol can be blamed for some of the world's most serious health problems. The less you drink the better" (*BMJ* 1994; 309: 1249).

The Royal Medical Colleges in Britain came out in strong support of the WHO, especially after a Danish group had suggested that drinking more than the recommended levels had a heart-protective effect: "Five pints a day keeps the doctor away," the Danes said. The Colleges warn that the INTERSALT study of over 10 000 people indicated an increased risk of haemorrhagic strokes at three or more units per day. They also warn that alcohol is implicated in 20% of cases of child abuse, 40% of road accidents and 39% of deaths in fires. One head of department states, "There has been wide coverage of how good alcohol is against heart disease without the coverage of how it increases wife battering and falls from building sites" (*BMJ* 1995; 310: 1623).

Nevertheless, despite the warnings, the British Government increased the limits for sensible drinking from three to four units per day for men and from two to three units per day for women, despite widespread criticism, including from the British Medical Association (*BMJ* 1996; 312: 7-9). Of course, individual alcohol intake varies considerably. Statistics indicate that 20% of people drink 80% of the alcohol in Britain, while a zealous 3% of drinkers knock off 30% of the stuff.

At present there is a worldwide tendency (including in Britain) to lower the legal limit of alcohol concentration of 80 mg per 100 ml (0.08%) to 50 mg per 100 ml (0.05%) for drivers. The Netherlands, France and Australia have already accepted the 0.05% legal level for driving. Sentences for exceeding these limits have become extremely severe.

However, researchers still continue to claim benefits for the heart from alcohol, much to the delight of the liquor trade. It is stated that alcohol may in part explain the French paradox of low heart-death rate in a Westernised society. But other factors that can cause this "paradox" are a high fresh fruit and vegetable intake, smaller meals (one seldom sees a fat French person), whole-wheat French loaves and a high butter/margarine intake ratio (70.6%/29.4%).

Despite an article which states that red wine increases the antioxidant activity in serum (*Lancet* 1994; 344: 193-4), it does appear that all types of alcoholic drinks are linked to a lower risk of heart attacks (*BMJ* 1996; 312: 731-6).

Of course, heart disease is not the only condition with a link to alcohol. The most common form of liver disease in the USA is related to alcoholism. All these cases have a history of five to 15 years of chronic alcohol intake (*Textbook of the Principles and Practice of Medicine*, 22nd edition, 1988). Another growing concern with increased alcohol intake is the increasing incidence of pancreatic cancer, even with mild but regular drinking.

The author has many times wondered which is the bigger evil, smoking or alcoholism. An Australian study, from the viewpoint of loss of time from work, indicated sick leave from smoking complications were estimated at an annual cost of 16.5 million dollars, as compared to alcohol at 5.5 million dollars. Smoking and alcoholism were together responsible for one-quarter of all sick leave from work (*Med J Australia* 1994; 161: 407-11). However, taking into consideration vehicle accidents, murders, assaults and child abuse, alcoholism appears to be the greater evil, by a slight margin.

The most effective therapy for alcoholism is through the world-wide organisation known as Alcoholics Anonymous (AA). The alcoholic only listens to one who has undergone the same problem, and can therefore talk his language. The AA also provides programmes for the family and friends of the alcoholic.

It should be remembered that alcohol also infiltrates the organs and tissues of the body, thereby negatively affecting the functions of micronutrients. The answer is to stay well within your capacity for alcohol, and if you are an abstainer, little advantage will be derived from starting on alcohol.

Exercise

A large number of studies have included exercise as part of their investigations. All agree that exercise in some form is necessary for good health. In the large nurses' study in the USA (*Lancet* 1993; 341: 581-85) vigorous physical activity, however, did not lessen the risk of heart attacks.

Let it be stressed that exercise must not be substituted for a correct diet. Suggestions such as, "I will neutralise this meal with a session in the gym later today", have no benefit. Doubt has been widely expressed concerning the effect of exercise alone, especially in regular gym workouts or daily running (jogging). In many cases this may be more useful to the bank accounts of orthopaedic surgeons than to the participant. In Sweden former athletes had 4.5 times the average risk of eventually needing a hip joint replacement for osteoarthritis. Those whose work had also exposed their joints to heavy loads had a relative risk of 8.5 (*Am J Sports Med* 1993; 21: 195-200).

It is also important that exercise should be enjoyable. The painful facial expressions on some joggers' faces are signs of defeated efforts and ambitions. Do not allow exercise to become an exasperating addiction, a well-recognised condition due to the secretion of habitual abnormal hormones in the brain known as endorphins. These alarmclock-like substances initiate a time factor that alerts the jogger to prepare for his regular daily run at the same time every day. No benefit is derived from such a procedure.

The British Cardiac Society Working Group, convened by Prof Michael Oliver (1987) clearly states that "physical activity should be encouraged as a normal part of daily living". Arguments that Western diseases, including heart disease, were absent in our forefathers' days due to their physical activity, is only true to a negligible extent. Our forefathers' natural high micronutrient diet was far more important.

The following suggestions are practical:
1. Be physically active as much as possible.
2. Take daily walks at a pace somewhere between enjoyment and effort. Change the locality of your walks from time to time, and seek pleasant surroundings and companions.
3. Sporting activities must be regular and well within the participant's physical ability.
4. Never use the lift if you can climb stairs.
5. Never drive if you can reasonably walk to your destination.

Relaxation

Relaxation's target is to lessen stress. The emotions and behaviour associated with stress are intense anxiety, depression, feelings of helplessness, and a type A behaviour, characterised by competitiveness, ambition, impatience and a sense of urgency.

It is far more practical to integrate relaxation into daily life. The following suggestions are applicable:
1. Find another legitimate interest or hobby outside the normal daily rou-

tine, for example woodwork, gardening in various forms, bird-watching, art, pottery, gem-grinding or -polishing, model-building.
2. Take an interest in some social activity which is useful to the community, such as antidrug abuse, feeding programmes for the needy, education, school programmes.
3. Music soothes the savage breast. Relax with your preferred music at home and in your car, taking care to avoid music that irritates. When opportune, attempt to take a short nap during the day, for example, after lunch. The nap should not last longer than ten to fifteen minutes. Participate in enjoyable exercise (see under Exercise).
4. Adopt a friendly attitude to everyone, even those you do not like, and clear up any misunderstandings you may have with people. Spend more time with your family and good friends, especially over weekends and holidays.
5. Always be active in mind and body in a positive sense, and avoid spending too much time contemplating the negative.

The Effect of a Correct Lifestyle on Disease

The effect of an improved lifestyle, similar to that of our forefathers before 1880, should make itself felt in health care, especially concerning Western diseases. This means a return to the genetic micronutrient diets, no smoking, controlled alcohol intake, less stress (later it will be shown that micronutrient shortages can have adverse effects on mood), and increased physical activity.

Is improvement in health possible without drugs and surgery? Results from the Lifestyle Heart Trial leave little doubt as to this possibility. To quote from the article, "Comprehensive lifestyle changes may be able to bring about regression (improved, return to normal) of even severe coronary atherosclerosis after only one year, without use of lipid-lowering drugs." Granted that the diet proposed in the article was a low-fat vegetarian diet (cholesterol intake was limited to 5 mg per day or less), which is certainly not a genetic micronutrient diet, the results nevertheless point to a totally new, inexpensive and effective treatment for atherosclerosis. Common sense dictates that this treatment will also be effective for other metabolic diseases. What the long-term effect of the above trial's specific diet will be on other disease states, has still to be determined.

Prof Alexander Leaf, Director of the Cardiovascular Health Centre at Boston, Massachusetts General Hospital and Harvard Professor of Preventative Medicine, stated, with reference to the above study, "This is going to shake up a lot of thinking." Prof Dean Ornish of the University of California, San Francisco, stated that the patient who showed the most improvement was the oldest, a 74-year-old man.

Consequently, there is an excellent outlook for everybody for whatever modern metabolic disease is present, and at any age.

CHAPTER 7

THE GENETIC MICRONUTRIENT DIET

One of the first duties of the physician is to advocate the masses not to take medicine.
SIR WILLIAM OSLER

The Basic Elements of the Micronutrient Diet

These basic elements have already been elaborated upon in the earlier chapters, but need to be re-emphasised here. The factors that play a role here are: the re-establishment of the lost micronutrients (vitamins and minerals); the recognition of different genetic races due to diet and climate; the recognition of probably all approximately 2 500 enzymes requiring micronutrients (one to five) in metabolic pathways; the knowledge that nearly a third of the enzymes and genes are polymorphic; and that virtually all metabolic diseases were either absent or rare before refinement of food in 1880.

This requires the recognition of 13 basic genetic diets, but as some of the 13 genetic races are small and, through emigration and intermarriage have even partly disappeared, not all the different diets will be discussed. The main diet will be directed at the North-West European descendents, the genetic race that has probably emigrated the most, but reference will be made to the Mediterraneans, the Africans, the Indo-Dravidians and the Sino-Japanese (Orientals). The other large group, the Central-East European, differs insignificantly from its North-Western cousins, and only individual points of difference will be touched upon.

A reminder is necessary regarding the methionine-homocysteine pathway, requiring the four micronutrients, vitamin B6, folic acid, vitamin B12 and magnesium, as well as the essential fatty acid-prostaglandin-thromboxane-leukotriene pathway, requiring the micronutrients vitamin B6, vitamin C, zinc, magnesium and nicotinic acid (niacin). The former plays a decisive role in coronary heart disease, venous thrombosis of the legs and strokes in the brain, while the latter, controlling the major physiological body functions, in its failure leads to the other major metabolic diseases, high blood pressure, diabetes mellitus type II, rheumatoid arthritis, cancer, osteoporosis, obesity, diverticulitis, spastic colon, depression, acne, auto-immune diseases, allergies, dental caries, and others.

The Basic Rules Applicable to the Genetic Micronutrient Diet (GMD)

Only two very basic rules have to be applied:

Firstly, the food in the diet must be as unrefined and unprocessed as possible, similar to the diets of genetic races before the advent of roller mills, canning, refrigeration and additives.

Secondly, the diet must be applicable to the genetic race of the individual.

A tragic example of where the two above-mentioned basic rules were not applied, due to circumstances beyond control, is described by Paul Herrman in his book *Sieben Vorbei und Acht verweht*, 1952. In 1921 excavations in Greenland revealed well-preserved bodies in the burial sites of a 14th-century Viking settlement. These tall, well-built emigrants from Norway landed, as a result of unplanned circumstances, among a community of Eskimos. Evidence indicates that the whole Viking community, which never intermarried with the Eskimos, died out within three generations. The later generations' bodies were found to suffer from severe abnormalities of bone, tuberculosis and rickets, and they had a much smaller build than the first generation. The main cause of the disaster was blamed on a change of diet, as their original provisions had run out and could not be replenished.

Problems in Applying the Genetic Micronutrient Diet (GMD)

The major problem we have in applying this diet is the fact that most of the foods that our forefathers enjoyed before the advent of roller mills (1880-1890) are no longer available. To whom should we address this problem? The food manufacturers have traditionally responded only to what the consumer wants. So it is obvious where the pressure must be applied. There is no reason why the manufacturers should not be able to supply products approximating as closely as possible to that enjoyed by our forefathers.

It is the consumer's duty to demand healthier food. Without consumer pressure the food manufacturer will not respond. The author has noted that in some food factories many employees are well aware of their own healthier unrefined products and personally consume it exclusively, even when that particular product is less than 1% of the factory's total output. If the consumer does not know the health facts no one in the factory's executive office is going to tell him, and thereby risk suffering a financial loss.

Much of the food produced today is geared to a longer shelf life. Gone are the days when farmers and many town dwellers baked their own daily bread from home-sifted flour, slaughtered their own livestock for the week's meat, or grew their own vegetables and fruit. Nowadays even the farmers buy nearly all their food from the supermarkets. Probably a certain percentage of micronutrient loss will never be regained by diet alone. Consequently, micronutrient supplementation will be necessary.

This supplementation can be applied in two ways. One is as a preventative against modern diseases, with a quantity added equal to the amount lost through food manufacture. Alternatively, once such diseases as atherosclerosis, high blood pressure, rheumatoid arthritis, etc. have become established, higher dosage supplementation is temporarily necessary, generally for one or two months. Even when additional conventional treatment has to be applied, experience has proved that added micronutrients will assist other forms of treatment to act more rapidly, effectively and over shorter periods.

Some will ask, "Why not remain on the old diet but just add micronutrients?" This is bad advice for two reasons. Firstly, the body has not been programmed to the processed foods, and the latter will still have grave effects on the body's metabolism. Secondly, micronutrients are, with very few exceptions such as in a slow-release form, not closely bound to the material binding the individual tablets, as in the case with natural foods. Consequently, micronutrients supplements will cause unnaturarally high blood levels immediately after dosage and then drop to below natural levels within two hours. This was established in our laboratories. In contrast, thanks to thousands of years of programming to maintain an optimum blood level during the course of the day, micronutrients in natural foods are released at a constant rate. It is therefore clear why a natural GM diet plus micronutrient supplementation are as near to the ideal as possible.

The Genetic Micronutrient (GM) Diet Proper

It will become clear that this basic diet is far easier to follow than any of the other prescribed diets, as for example the misnamed "prudent" diet of the American Heart Association – provided that the foods are readily available. It compares well with the eating habits of our forefathers. Although they did not follow any strict dietary rules, metabolic diseases, including heart attacks, were extremely rare. Their simple rule was to eat what was available, a rule if applied today would lead to disaster. What was available had been genetically programmed for thousands of years. The reason for their superb metabolic health was that their basic foods – bread, cereals, rice, meats, vegetables and fruits – were unrefined and unprocessed, thereby assuring them of an abundance of functional and protective micronutrients.

The general rules of the GM diet are as follows:
1. Include as much as possible of unrefined and unprocessed foods.
2. Where possible avoid canned or frozen foods. This is not always practical but do your best.
3. Recognise your own genetic race and follow its genetic diet.
4. Vary the genetic diet to counter monotony. The choice is wide.
5. The less you eat without starving or damaging your health, the better.
6. For an ordinary working day, have a substantial breakfast and only one other large meal per day.
7. Eat animal protein (red meat, fish or chicken) only once a day.
8. Establish this new diet as soon as possible and continue it for the rest of your life.

Breakfast or Morning Meal

For an ordinary working day, consider breakfast to be the most important meal of the day. Certainly do not omit or neglect it, a habit too prevalent amongst young persons. "Oh, I never have time for breakfast", is too much the call of a lazy, exhausted waster. A high micronutrient diet (which may coincide with the less important high energy content) will prime you for your whole working day.

It is customary to distinguish between a warm winter's and a cold summer's breakfast in your choice of cereals.

The warm winter's cereals are represented by maize (corn), oats and sorghum, or modifications thereof. It would be appropriate to look again at the relevant micronutrient content of these cereals (Table 7.1). Note partic-

	MAIZE SUPER mg%	MAIZE STRAIGHT-RUN RAW mg%	SORGHUM mg%	OATS BRAN RAW mg%
Magnesium	32	123	117	223
Zinc	0.50	2.30	2.64	2.96
Riboflavin	0.03	0.12	0.15	0.21
Niacin	0.60	2.20	3.90	0.90
Vit. B6	0.04	0.30	?	0.16
Folic Acid	14 (ug%)	33 (ug%)	?	49 (ug%)
Vit. C	0	0	0	0

Table 7.1. A comparison of three basic cereals and their micronutrient content, three unrefined examples compared to the most refined.

ularly the high micronutrient content of sorghum, oats and unrefined maize as compared to that of refined maize. This, however, still excludes the role of the genetic factors.

Maize (mealie meal, corn). Avoid the refined maize products (super and special) and use only unsifted whole kernel products. The latter have become extremely scarce, especially commercially. Approach the local maize mills for aid. Unfortunately, owing to the high germ-oil content, these products should be bought in small quantities and kept in a refrigerator. How our forefathers stored their maize is a mystery.

Oats. Long considered to be Scotland's breakfast gruel, oats in contrast with other cereals has been a disappointment in effectively lowering the blood cholesterol. Mixed and opposing results have been obtained in different studies (*NEJM* 1990; 322: 147-52).

Oats is a secondary crop from the primary grain crops, wheat and barley. The oldest reference to it is relatively recent, only 1000 BC in central Europe. Sheriff, a Scot farmer, was the first to start producing oats in Scotland on a large scale only in the 1860s (N.W. Simmonds, *Evolution of Crop Plants*, 1979). The belief that oats is the ancient food of the Scots is therefore incorrect, but it may have been that of the Central-East Europeans. The Scots are known to have a very high incidence of heart attack deaths. They would most probably regard it as sacrilege if it were suggested they go back to wheat and refrain from oats. However, they only have another eight centuries to go before oats becomes programmed to their diet, or that of all Sassenachs.

Scots also eat very little fruit and vegetables (personal note, Prof H Tunstall-Pedoe, Aberdeen, 1990). It would be reasonable to believe that the mixed results obtained with oats could be due to varied genetic races in the same studies.

Digestive bran. This previously considered waste from wheat flour contains 44% fibre and the highest combined concentrations of vitamin B6, zinc and magnesium of any food (Table 7.2). Add one to two tablespoons and mix it thoroughly with breakfast cereals, even before cooking if preferred. Usually bran is considered disposable and fed to pigs and cattle, allowing them an extremely healthy, if short-lived, existence. Regular amounts of natural digestive bran added to a balanced diet is probably the most reliable and healthy method of avoiding constipation. Always use the very inexpensive natural bran. It can also be used as an appetite suppressant half an hour before meals.

Summer cereals. Only those with the highest micronutrient and fibre content are recommended. These include All-Bran Flakes, Raisin Bran, Weetbix and the mueslis (see Appendix). The market is presently being flooded by

	WHEAT GERM	BRAN	WHOLE-WHEAT FLOUR 97%	BROWN BREAD FLOUR 86%	WHITE BREAD FLOUR 76%
Vitamin B6 mg/100g	1.15	1.38	0.18	0.10	0.04
Zinc mg/100g	14.30	16.20	2.32	2.11	1.80
Magnesium mg/100g	336.00	520.00	78.00	52.00	26.00
Fibre g/100g	20.30	44.00	8.90	5.30	2.80

Table 7.2. Illustrating the effect of bread preparation and refinement. Wheat flour is initially reduced to a 70% extraction, which is used for cake flour. Wheat germ and fibre are then separated from the rest of the flour. Bran is then added to the refined wheat flour corresponding to the necessary concentrations for white bread (76%) and brown bread (86%). Note that wheat germ is not returned to the bread flour. (Ref.: *Composition of Foods, Agricultural Handbook No 8*, 1975, 1984, USA.)

new health products and a wide variety is available. Give preference to the natural products and be careful of the synthetic fibre and added micronutrient brands.

Bread. This should be restricted to whole-wheat bread exclusively. Wheat bread is the staple food of 35% of the world population. In the preparation of bread the flour is first extracted to a 70% concentration. This is cake flour. At the same time the digestive bran and wheat germ bran are separated. Digestive bran is returned to the flour to establish the necessary concentrations needed, for example, for white (76%) and brown (86%) bread (Table 7.2.). Whole-wheat bread is, in fact, a misnomer, as the 3% wheat germ is never returned to the flour. Wheat germ contains a most nutritious natural oil which, unfortunately, decreases the shelf life of bread but contains a very large percentage of the antioxidants, vitamins A, D, E and beta-carotene, so vitally necessary for the body's normal metabolism. Little does the tradesman know that the longer the shelf life of his bread, the shorter the life of his client, and therefore in the long run he loses more than he gains.

Another problem has now been discovered with modern-day bread. Due to the propaganda which has encouraged the view that vegetable fats are advisable for health reasons, stabilisers used in bread-baking now contain these fats instead of the older animal fats. Consequently white bread (and cookies or biscuits) contain a high percentage of transfatty acids which, as we have shown, increase both blood cholesterol and the incidence of heart attacks (*Lancet* 1993; 341: 581-5).

Crisp breads (Ryvita, Provita, etc.) are acceptable as alternatives or additions to bread, especially in the treatment of obesity. A large percentage of people still eat white bread – the South African figures in 1985 were 45% of whites, 65% of coloureds and 10% of blacks (*Davin Report*).

Butter. This has been extensively discussed in Chapter 3. To repeat the important factors, all extensive studies comparing butter and margarine have unanimously reported that margarine, in all its forms, increases cholesterol and the incidence of heart attacks, whilst butter has no deleterious effects. Three factors probably play a role: an overdose of polyunsaturated fatty acids and abnormal transfatty acids in margarine, and a genetic programming of butter for a few thousand years. As in all cases, moderation is necessary. Claims that margarine can provide a transfatty-free product increases the price exhorbitantly but fails to address the overdose of PUFAs or the genetic factor. If the price of butter is still too high, rather exclude all fatty smears. Remember as well, that saturated fatty acids have now been proved not to increase the blood cholesterol.

Milk. The belief that the intake of full-cream milk should be restricted because of its incumbent cholesterol intake has been proved by various very reliable studies to be totally incorrect. An overzealous belief that all foods containing cholesterol are bad ignores the role of genetics, man's programmer over thousands of years. When four pints of fresh full-cream milk (just under two litres) were given to Cambridge volunteers daily for two weeks, their blood cholesterols decreased (Howard A.N. and Marks J., *Lancet*, 1977). But the most convincing evidence was in the halfway findings of the five-year Caerphilly study, 1991, where it was shown that of 164 men who drank more than one pint of full-cream milk a day only 1.2% had heart attacks, and of 162 men who drank no milk 9.9% had heart attacks. Skimmed milk should be restricted to those who are desperate to lose weight. The role of lactase enzymes in different races is a factor to contend with. It must be remembered that yoghurt is an artificially produced fermented milk, and can be produced from whole, low-fat or skim milk.

Beverages. Coffee or tea with or without full-cream milk and moderate sugar (one teaspoon) is totally acceptable. Coffee should be restricted only if a person has abnormal heart palpitations, and caffeine content is a matter of choice. Coffee causing an increase in blood lipids is so insignificant that it can be ignored. Herbal tea's only advantage above ordinary tea is that it has no caffeine. Five or six cups of coffee or tea should be the average. Fresh fruit drinks are highly recommended.

Fruit. Choose from any available fruits, but take into consideration the micronutrient content according to the appendix tables. Note particularly the high content in bananas (the tennis champions' favourite, and for a very good reason), avocados (it is still controversial whether it increases weight), kiwis and figs. Stewed fruits and unsweetened fruit rolls are recommended. Beware of too high a fruit intake, it could resemble a spastic colon with diarrhoea.

Eggs. All studies, without exception, have shown that two whole eggs per day in a balanced diet does not affect the blood cholesterol levels. Remember, all races of man have eaten eggs for thousands of years. William Connor of the USA has for years been the spokesman for the American Heart Association, advancing the cholesterol-increasing effect of eggs. However, in every one of his published experiments he used only the yolks of eggs. This is certainly not the way an egg is normally eaten. Prof Estie Vorster of Potchefstroom, South Africa, proved that in students it made no difference whether they ate three, seven or fourteen eggs per week, their blood cholesterol values remained unchanged. An experiment on male students by the author has shown that the manner in which eggs are prepared may play a role. Two boiled eggs per day for two months given in addition to the normal diet, lowered the cholesterol, whereas fried eggs given to three groups, one prepared in butter, one in vegetable oils and one in margarine, all increased the blood cholesterol. Consequently boiled, or poached, or scrambled eggs or omelettes prepared in Teflon pans (with no butter, oil or margarine) can reasonably be considered harmless and, of course, highly nutritious. The original recommendation to restrict eggs to two a week to remain within the 300 mg daily cholesterol intake, and its later modification to four eggs per week, by the AHA and the Heart Foundations, has no experimental support and is totally unfounded.

Spreads. Marmite, Fray Bentos and Bovril are recommended.

Summary

The following examples of breakfast are recommended, but each person can improvise within the basic laws of the genetic micronutrient diet. The important items are in bold letters.

1. **Unrefined maize cereal** with 1-2 tablespoons of **digestive bran** stirred in, honey or minimum sugar, whole milk; one cup of tea or coffee with full-cream milk and sweeteners; one **banana**.
2. A bowl of **Weet-Bix**, **Hi-Bulk Bran** or **mueslis** or any other genuine **unrefined breakfast cereal** (study the content labels carefully), or a mixture of the above, plus **digestive bran**, with whole milk, minimum sugar or honey; **stewed fruit** or **fresh fruit**; one cup of tea or coffee with full-cream milk and sweeteners.
3. One or two **boiled** or **poached eggs**, or an omelette prepared in a Teflon

pan; one to two slices of **whole-wheat bread** (plain or toasted) with **butter** and **Marmite, Fray Bentos** or **Bovril**; **stewed fruit** or **fresh fruit** or a **fruit drink**.

The following advice is directed at various genetic races.

Africans: They should have unrefined sorghum (unfortunately extremely difficult to obtain), fermented or fresh milk, a minimum amount of sugar or honey, tea or coffee with milk as mentioned before, minimum sugar and/or a fruit.

Indo-Dravidians: They should have substantially unrefined breads and biscuits. Cereals are not customary but teas are. Breakfast is traditionally a small meal, and for genetic reasons it may remain so. Religious restrictions are to be obeyed, especially as they have been part of the diet for many generations.

Sino-Japanese: They should increase the amount of breakfast with choices of fish, eggs (boiled), fruit (especially kumquat), or dumpling bread containing meat (pork, lamb, goat, poultry). Further, traditional teas.

Mediterraneans: They should stick to their traditional unrefined breads, fruit (grapes, apricots, dates, figs, melons, plums, peaches, pears, quinces, raisins) and cheeses (traditional and minimally processed). The cereals and bread must be unrefined. Coffee is preferred to tea.

The Midday Meal

The habit of eating three meals a day can be dated back to the ancient Greeks and Romans (Ken McGleich, *Food and drink: Greeks and Romans*). Few Greek or Roman women were active breadwinners, so meals could be prepared three times a day. In modern times this custom has changed considerably. Consequently it is the custom that, apart from breakfast, one of the two remaining meals should be small and the other a major one.

From a health point of view there is no danger in cutting down or even omitting one meal a day, provided breakfast is adequate. Modern convention has it that the midday meal or lunch must, for the day worker, be the smaller one. A big danger lies in too many modern executive lunches.

For practical reasons the midday meal will be discussed here as the lighter one, but this could be reversed, as over weekends.

Sandwiches: Whole-wheat or crisp bread (Ryvita, Provita), with or without butter. Smears of Marmite, Fray Bentos, Bovril or similar natural extracts.

Salads: Note the list in the appendix. Fresh spinach should be sliced and eaten raw. Add beetroot, potato, green beans, carrots, cabbage, cauliflower, peppers, asparagus, mushrooms or tomato (the latter for vitamin C). Note the low micronutrient content in cucumbers and lettuce, both of doubtful nutritional value.

Fruit and fruit drinks: As for breakfast.

Important: Skip animal protein (meat, fish, chicken) if the evening meal will contain it.

Business lunches: This can be any businessman's stairway to heaven . . . via a heart attack through overindulgence. If ever a meal can kill, it will be this one, especially if it is accompanied or followed by a stressful meeting.

Vegetable oils: If used, go for the more natural pressed oils, rare and expensive. All oils should be used only once and then discarded. Re-use will increase the danger of transfatty acid formation. Good advice is to restrict vegetable oils to sprinkling over salads.

Mayonnaise: Restrict to salads as an alternative to vegetable oils. It has a high PUFA content, now known to have an unhealthy effect.

Cheese: This is as old a food as butter and milk. Owing to its high cholesterol content the AHA has given it a bad name, which is, as with butter and milk, entirely unjustified. Cheese was a major dietary food in the ancient Roman and Greek diets (Ken McGleish, ibid.). As expected, preference should be given to the more ancient and natural cheeses, such as cottage, cheddar, Edam, Gouda and Swiss. As with all good foods, do not overindulge. It may be advisable, as has been suggested, that not more than what fits into a standard matchbox should be eaten per day.

Summary

To summarise, the following choices of menus are acceptable with the important items in bold print.

1. One or two **whole-wheat sandwiches** (or **whole-wheat buns**) with **butter** and Fray Bentos; an **apple**, **banana** or **orange;** and a pure **fruit beverage.**
2. Salad dish (**cabbage, sliced raw spinach, carrots, tomatoes,** asparagus, mushrooms) with vegetable oils or mayonaise; **cheese** (cottage, cheddar, Edam, Gouda, Swiss); cup of coffee or tea with milk and sweeteners.
3. Executive lunch: fruit or fish as hors d'oeuvre; fillet of beef steak (or steamed fish); salad mixture as above; vegetables (**spinach, potato-in-skin, peas, beans, cabbage, cauliflower**); **fruit salad;** coffee or tea. Remember to have only a light meal the same evening.

In most other genetic races the afternoon and evening meals do not differ that much, so the following descriptions cover both meals.

Africans: Whole-wheat sandwiches (never white bread), fermented milk, fruit (bananas, apple, or orange), vegetables (cabbage, spinach or *marog*, jacket potatoes, pumpkin and pumpkin seeds, maize-on-the-cob), beans (diynawa, samp-and-bean mixtures), unsalted peanuts, tea and coffee with minimum sugar, fermented milk.

Indo-Dravidians: Religious restrictions must be respected, particularly as, for health reasons, they may be part of the programming of enzymes and receptors. Otherwise pork, beef, chicken, sausages, oxtails, liver and stomach.

Also milk, frequently fermented, dates, honey, olive oil. Vegetables include pumpkin, spinach, bamboo shoots, mushrooms, squash, squash blossoms and young shoots, tomato, cabbage, watercress, cucumber, broccoli, carrots, cauliflower, nepa cabbage, mustard greens, bittermelon, watermelon, green beans, eggplant and water chestnut.

Rice is extremely important, constituting some 60% of the kilojoule intake, but exclusively unrefined or brown rice should be eaten. Vegetables should not be overcooked. Olive oil is okay, since it is genetically determined and programmed.

Fruits include bananas, mangoes, pawpaws, pineapples, melons, oranges and grapefruit.

Sino-Japanese: Rice is the main food, essentially brown or paddy, also barley, oats and rye. Fish is another staple food, but should be only moderately salted to avoid the danger of stomach cancer.

Meat includes pork (the favourite), lamb, goat and poultry. Beef is being increasingly eaten by the Japanese. This is not wise for genetic reasons as there is a danger of increasing heart disease and cancer.

Soya bean products are genetically programmed to Sino-Japanese, provided they are unrefined and natural.

Vegetables include carrots, onions, leeks, peas, cabbages, turnips, cucumbers, beans, squash, sprouts and sweet potatoes. The main oil is peanut oil, but soya oils and rice oils are also used and acceptable.

Mediterraneans: Their main dish is vegetables, boiled or fried in olive oil. These include cabbage, cauliflower, cucumbers, eggplant, greens, okra, onions, peppers, potatoes, vine leaves, tomatoes and solid greens. Fruits include oranges, lemons and grapes, usually eaten raw.

Maize and rice are not common cereals, but bread is popular and should be unrefined. Pasta is traditional and genetic, supposed to have been introduced by Marco Polo from China since early in the thirteenth century, but others believe it could have been earlier.

Lamb is the main meat, with beef, goat, mutton, pork and poultry eaten less often.

Fish is commonly eaten. Eggs are popular as also are white beans and legumes. Cheeses have traditionally been widely used. The main oil is olive oil. Coffee and wine are popular beverages.

The Evening Meal

This will be considered as the large or main meal of the day. The advisability of having a large meal in the evening is debatable on grounds of a full stomach at night. The criticism is valid, but modern convention has it that most Westerners work a daylight eight-hour session or more away from home. Consequently a large home-cooked meal is out of the question. Weekends are a different matter and then the larger midday meals are the custom.

Red meat (or beef). The AHA and heart foundations have given this commodity a bad name, which is highly unjustified. Too much meat may be a bad thing, but that goes for everything. Most of the criticism is aimed at red meat's supposedly high cholesterol and saturated fat content, and their recommendations are rather to eat fish and chicken. Table 7.3 reveals the misrepresentation of their statements that the fat *inside* the red meat has such a high cholesterol content as compared to fish and chicken, as for practical reasons it is the same in all three meats. Must we conclude from the AHA's statements that the cholesterol in red meat is bad for you, while the same concentration in fish and chicken is acceptable? Surely not!

The AHA further argues that the ratio of the type of fat is less favourable in red meat than in others. Mention has already been made in this book that increased polyunsaturated fats are a factor in a number of diseases such as cancer and allergies, while saturated fats have been proved not to increase the blood cholesterol. Table 7.3 also indicates the high micronutrient content of red meat, which is probably more important than the fats, at least in heart disease. Note the favourable micronutrient content in red meat compared to those in chicken, particularly the important blood-forming factors, vitamin B12 and iron.

Note too the very high content of the amino acid, methionine, in red meat, the highest in any food, and the forerunner of homocysteine, a factor found to be nearly eight times more of a risk for heart disease than blood cholesterol. Now it is reasonable to believe that the homocysteine concentration in red meat is far more of a factor in heart disease than blood cholesterol was ever supposed to be.

It is a well-known fact that nations with a high meat consumption (USA, Argentina, Australia, New Zealand, South Africa) have a high incidence of heart attack deaths, but this only became apparent after the 1920s. This was the time in dietary history when the loss of the protective effects of the micronutrients became effective.

	Meth-ionine	Chol (1)	Chol (2)	Tot Fat	Sat Fat	MUFA	PUFA
	mg/100 g			g/100 g			
Meat, beef, lean	0.888	82	83	7.4	3.04	3.44	0.29
Meat, beef, with fat	0.888	82	83	14.0	6.25	7.07	0.60
Lamb, lean	0.410	110	93	12.3	5.99	4.66	0.58
Chicken, no skin	0.537	83	83	6.7	1.84	2.39	1.54
Fish, cod	0.480	80	60	3.7	0.99	0.55	0.13
Sausage, pork	0.228	83	83	31.2	10.81	13.90	3.81

	Mg	Zn	B6	Fe	B12
	mg/100 g				g/100 g
Beef, grilled, lean	22	5.5	0.33	3.8	2.65
Beef, grilled, with fat	24	5.3	0.29	3.1	2.65
Lamb, lean	28	5.3	0.22	2.2	?
Chicken, no skin	21	1.99	0.26	1.2	0.42
Fish, steamed	15	0.55	0.83	1.1	0.60

Table 7.3. A comparison of methionine (the important amino acid in the diet forming homocysteine), cholesterol, fatty acids, and micronutrients in animal fats. Two different sources are quoted: 1.) *Composition of Foods, Agricultural Handbook, USA, 1975*; 2.) *Nutritive Value of Foods, Home and Garden Bulletin Number 72*, US Department of Agriculture, 1981. Note particularly the similar cholesterol content of cholesterol in all animal fats, and the large differences in zinc, iron, and vitamin B12 content.

Prof W.C. Willett and his co-workers at Harvard Medical School have indicated that red meat is a factor in colon cancer in women but not in heart attacks (*NEJM* 1990; 323: 1664-72). Could it be that the genetic factors, which were not considered in this study, may play a role in the above results?

The following points are therefore significant:
1. Animal fat intake, including that of red meat, varied from genetic race to genetic race over thousands of years. Consequently dietary advice on meat should vary according to genetic race history.
2. Those nations (not necessarily races) with a high red meat consumption (sometimes with all three daily meals as in the not-too-distant past) have among the highest heart attack death rates, but this only

became apparent after the protective effects of dietary micronutrients were lost.
3. Although a high red meat diet, without micronutrients from other sources (B6, zinc, magnesium, folate, vitamin B12, vitamin C) could lead to heart attacks, the alternative of a too low or no red meat diet could lead to other micronutrient losses (iron, vitamin B12, folate) with the development of a troublesome anaemia.

A compromise is therefore necessary to meet the computerised needs of man's metabolism.

Fish: The main advantage of fish is that it contains oils which form the prostaglandin 3 series. This is far more important than its supposedly low cholesterol intake (which is not obvious), or its supposedly favourable fatty-acid composition. Genetics also play an important role here, and the genetic fish-eating races should remain on high fish diets. Fish oil capsules are expensive, but as little as two fish dishes per week have been shown to be effective in treating atherosclerosis in Dutch men (Kromhout D., *NEJM*, 1985). In a study of 2 033 male survivors of heart attacks, fatty fish reduced the overall deaths by 27% and deaths from heart attacks by one-third (*Lancet* 1992; ii: 757-61).

Chicken: Being considered a later addition to the genetic diet of man than red meat and fish, this commodity has little health advantage above the other two. Price is its main advantage. It has been stated that the skin should be removed because of its high cholesterol content, but this advice has been challenged lately.

Practical Advice on Animal fats: In genetic races of North-West European origin restrict animal fats to only one meal per day. A practical suggestion would be twice a week fish, with red meat and chicken distributed between the other days. Only sausages prepared from lean meat should be used. Beware of a too-high salt content in dried meat (South Africa: biltong) and limit its intake. Regarding barbecues, give preference to the Chinese (Mongolian) type, with lean meat, raw vegetables and butter or fresh oils, prepared in a wok. Avoid extended boiling in iron pots, for it destroys nearly all the vitamins. To be strictly avoided are all processed meats, such as polony, viennas and salami, etc. Rare animal foods, such as caviar, bone marrow, shrimps, liver, kidneys, etc. should be sparingly partaken of, to save both your health and, in some cases, your purse.

Vegetables: Note the list in the appendix. Always prepare moderately raw. In rough order of preference, according to micronutrient content, the following: spinach, peas, potato in skin, green beans, carrots, cabbage, cauliflower, Brussels sprouts, brinjals, sweet potatoes, squash, onions. Where a choice exists, give preference to fresh vegetables rather than frozen.

Rice: The oldest reference to rice in the world dates back to 3500 BC in Thailand. Later dates are 3280-2750 BC in China and 2500 BC in India. It is a well-documented fact that Indians emigrating to England, Trinidad and South Africa develop an extremely high incidence of Western diseases, including diabetes, heart attacks and high blood pressure. These immigrants also acquire a greater body mass index, higher blood cholesterols, higher apolipoprotein B and lower HDL-cholesterol (*Lancet* 1995; 345: 405-9). It all correlates well with a higher fat and cholesterol intake, but the question arises, "How much could be due to a changed white rice diet?" The same rule applies to Japanese immigrants to San Francisco and Hawaii. The recommendation is, therefore, to eat exclusively brown rice. To examplify, white rice has lost 93% of its most important mineral, magnesium, compared to brown rice.

Further General Dietary Recommendations

Salt: Table salt (NaCl) should be severely restricted, and if possible substituted by multiple micronutrient salts. Salt restriction has had surprising results, as when in the USA some years ago it was publicly propagated. The change had little effect on high blood pressure, but dramatically curtailed gastric cancer.

In-betweens: Crisp breads with tasty natural spreads.

Alcohol: This has been fully discussed in the previous chapter.

Nonalcoholic drinks: Give preference to fresh fruit drinks.

Confectionery: Restrict severely. Unsugared and dried fruits are recommended. Cakes and biscuits should be prepared from unrefined flour.

Hamburgers: "A teenager's idea of a balanced diet is a hamburger in each hand." This very common food commodity is the cause of much of the modern metabolic diseases, with its abnormal transfatty acid content of both white bread and vegetable oils plus processed meat. Yet it would make literally a world of change if whole-wheat rolls were universally used plus butter and lean meat.

Dried potato chips: Prepared in boiling vegetable oils, this commodity's danger is the high concentration of abnormal transfatty acids present. Boiling continues for 72 hours, so a variation in harmful transfatty acid concentration occurs, lower at the start and much higher towards the end (Enig M.G. et al., *JAOCS* 1983; 60: 1788-95). The packaging fails to mention this, so go slow on chips.

Pastas: This traditional Mediterranean food has been said to have been introduced by Marco Polo from China in the early 1300s, but other sources believe it to be earlier. Few studies, if any, have included pastas in their data, but genetically it may be a factor in Western diseases.

Garlic: This malodorous plant has actually been proved to have various beneficial effects on heart disease. Garlic powder, 600-900 mg per day, reduced total blood cholesterol by 8-12%, probably through inhibition of cholesterol formation and antioxidant acivity. It lowered blood pressure through dilating the blood vessels. Furthermore it reduced plasma viscosity and platelet aggregation, increased blood flow and increased breakdown of fibrin clots. Is this the "Mediterranean connection"? (*Atherosclerosis X*, Oct. 1994).

Sugar: Use strictly in moderation, never more than one teaspoon per cup, or use sweeteners. The micronutrient content of brown and white sugar differ insignificantly. Honey is an excellent replacement.

Soy Protein: This food has been advocated frequently as being cholesterol-lowering and as a replacement for red meat (*NEJM* 1995; 333: 313-4). However, genetically it is only acceptable to Asian populations. Soy contains oestrogens and is said to cause a decline in male sperm counts (*NEJM* 1995; 333: 276-82).

Warning: Initially the GM diet may cause flatulence or heartburn, due to the new high fibre content. This is temporary, but may take quite a time to disappear completely in sensitive patients.

Final Note on the GM Diet

This is not a difficult diet to follow. The biggest problem is the unavailability of the original foods. The positive effect may not be felt immediately as the body tissues, having suffered severe shortages of micronutrients for a long period of time, must now gradually re-establish the biochemical reactions to their optimum effect.

Health advice all over the world is steadily moving in the direction of genetic micronutrient diet and supplementation. Expressions such as "natural" and "traditional" are now common. However, beware of "natural" foods which are not genetically determined by race.

Experiences of our forefathers some three to four generations back, suggest that a temporary digression in the diet may be allowed. However, do not be too lax or overdo it. The Western disease that you have been cured of may return abruptly.

A specific diet for those who wish to decrease their mass will be discussed under the heading **Obesity** in Chapter 9.

In practice a comparison of some micronutrients (vitamin B6, magnesium, zinc) can be made between a conventional daily diet and a high micronutrient diet. A conventional breakfast of two fried eggs and bacon, one slice of white toast and margarine, a small dish of super maize, skimmed milk and coffee, a midday meal of two white sandwiches with margarine and one orange, and an evening meal of chicken 100 grams, five vegetables (beans, pumpkin, onion, turnips, white rice) and baked pudding, will contain approximately 0.9 mg vitamin B6, 170 mg magnesium and 6 mg zinc. A day's intake of two boiled eggs, unrefined maize and whole-cream milk, two tablespoons of bran, one slice of whole-wheat bread with butter, a fruit cocktail, a midday meal of two whole-wheat sandwiches, butter and two bananas, and an evening meal of 100 g beef with selected vegetables (potato, cabbage, cauliflower, spinach, brown rice), plus fruit salad, will yield approximately 4.5 mg vitamin B6, 600 mg magnesium and 18 mg zinc. The difference is approximately 5 times higher vitamin B6, and 3 times higher magnesium and zinc in the latter diet than in the former.

Aldous Huxley once said, "Facts do not cease to exist because they are ignored."

Common Subterfuges Regarding the Diet

After many years of offering advice on the genetic micronutrient diet, the following subterfuges and excuses from individuals have been encountered. The general appropriate responses are added.

"I don't care for the diet."
Then you haven't tried the "prudent diet" of the American Heart Association. This is far more tasteful and acceptable than that, and your forefathers lived on it for hundreds of years. Your tastebuds have been indoctrinated for too long by the food manufacturers' refined products. In 60% of coronary heart cases the patients also did not care for it, but they found it most palatable after their first coronaries. The other 40% had no choice: they all died.

"Bran tastes like sawdust."
The pigs don't think so. Don't eat or drink it as such. Either mix it in a fruit drink or mix it in a breakfast food, and add milk and sugar in moderate amounts.

"I can't spread butter. It is too hard."
Your grandmother never complained. Take a little out and place it on top of the fridge. Butter scrapers are inexpensive tools. Do not mix it with other vegetable oils, the latter have been proved injurious to your health by lowering your resistance to diseases such as asthma and other allergies.

"Whole-wheat bread doesn't cut easily and it crumbles in the breadcutter."
Bakers have problems with whole-wheat bread baking and tend to neglect the finer details. Look for the home-baked type and shop around. Your grandmother had no problems and neither did the millions before her. Of course they had no choice. The average intake of bread in England at the turn of the century was three-quarters of a loaf a day.

"The roughage blows me up and I pass more winds."
This is a very common complaint at the start and it may last quite a time, but it is entirely due to the bran fibre, so reintroduce it gradually. It will eventually pass – I mean, go away.

"My bowels act more frequently."
And your stools are softer, so be thankful. Once more it is due to the fibre, and if you continue you will never become constipated again. It is to your health's advantage. In Hippocrates' time daily stools occurred two to three times a day.

"I have a spastic colon and my doctor says I may not eat any roughage."
Your doctor is old-fashioned, or incorrectly informed. It was because you ate no roughage that you developed a spastic colon. Follow the diet and you will notice the disappearance, at least partially, of your condition.

"I cannot eat any carbohydrates because I am a diabetic."
Carbohydrates can either be refined as in sugars, or unrefined or complex as in grains. The former is not allowed, but the latter is obligatory as it contains all the micronutrients necessary to battle against diabetes and keep blood sugars low.

"I don't like spinach."
Then eat it raw as a salad; slice it and add a salad dressing.

"Brown rice takes too long to cook."
You should really weigh up this short extra cooking time against an increased proclivity towards atherosclerosis, high blood pressure and diabetes.

"I have a sweet tooth for chocolates and cake."
First take a good look at your figure in the mirror, then apply your willpower to restrict such indulgences to the absolute minimum. If your resistance collapses, restrict yourself to black or bitter chocolate. It is made from cocoa and has a very high magnesium content.

"I take three or four whiskys a day, and my friends have many more beers. Besides, the French have lots more wine than two glasses a day and they have a low incidence of heart attacks."
You are really playing with fire, risking not only a high possibility of chronic alcoholism, but also the healthy functioning of your liver. You have a strong possibility of developing liver cirrhosis within ten years. The French paradox is not only due to alcohol. They also have a high intake of fruit and vegetables. Furthermore they are the country with the lowest margarine intake in the world. Incidentally, the French are known for their high incidence of liver cancer and cirrhosis. So take your pick.

"I am allergic to certain vitamins and minerals."
You are unique, so unique that I would advise a reinvestigation. This could be due to other ingredients in the pills used. Change your origin of medication.

"I don't need a diet because I am taking high dosages of vitamins and minerals."
You are excreting an extremely precious form of urine and faeces; it is an absolute shame that such valuable excreta should be lost to the pharmaceutical industry. There are no particular advantages and possibly some disadvantages attached to taking unnecessarily high dosages of vitamins and minerals, especially when they are not taken in the natural slow-release form. Nature has exclusively developed such a natural slow-release form and we should adhere to it as closely as possible. You are also not taking your genetic diet into consideration, which is at least half the battle.

"Vitamins and minerals make you fat."
Quite the opposite. In stimulating the complete metabolism the body tends towards a loss of weight.

CHAPTER 8

THE OTHER GREATER METABOLIC DISEASES

Research is to see what everybody else has seen, and to think what nobody else has thought.
ALBERT SZENT-GYÖRGYI

Introduction

Although heart disease is the late 20th-century's greatest killer in the developed world, there is every reason to believe that it is only the spearhead of a list of metabolic diseases, reminiscent of a stampeding crowd of animals, following their leader in a destructive drive to flatten all before them. If this is true, what is the stimulus that initiated it all? Common factors of time, incidents and stimuli would be of paramount importance. And lo and behold, we have every reason to believe that those very factors are screaming at us for recognition.

By this chapter the reader should be only too aware of those damning factors that play such a devastating role in man's health — the loss of micronutrients through food-processing procedures. Since 1880, this constant and increasing loss has insidiously gnawed away at our delicately balanced metabolism to produce diseases that were virtually unheard of a century ago. Succumbing to well-organised commercial interests, we glut our bodies and metabolic pathways with half-measures and "quarter-effects" that inflict pernicious damage on our bodily mechanisms.

Though many metabolic pathways are obviously affected by the micronutrient losses, it would appear that the methionine-homocysteine and the essential fatty-acid-prostaglandin pathways play a critical role in the development of modern metabolic diseases. Fig 8.1. demonstrates figuratively how this pathology is developed. Although the mentioned micronutrients play a highly important role, it must be realised that other micronutrients, playing perhaps a lesser role, are nonetheless absolutely necessary to many normal metabolic pathways.

The author has a problem in deciding which are "the other greater metabolic diseases" in comparison to "the other lesser metabolic diseases", and to a certain degree this is a personal choice with which other experts in this field may differ. No disease is greater than any sufferer's present ailment.

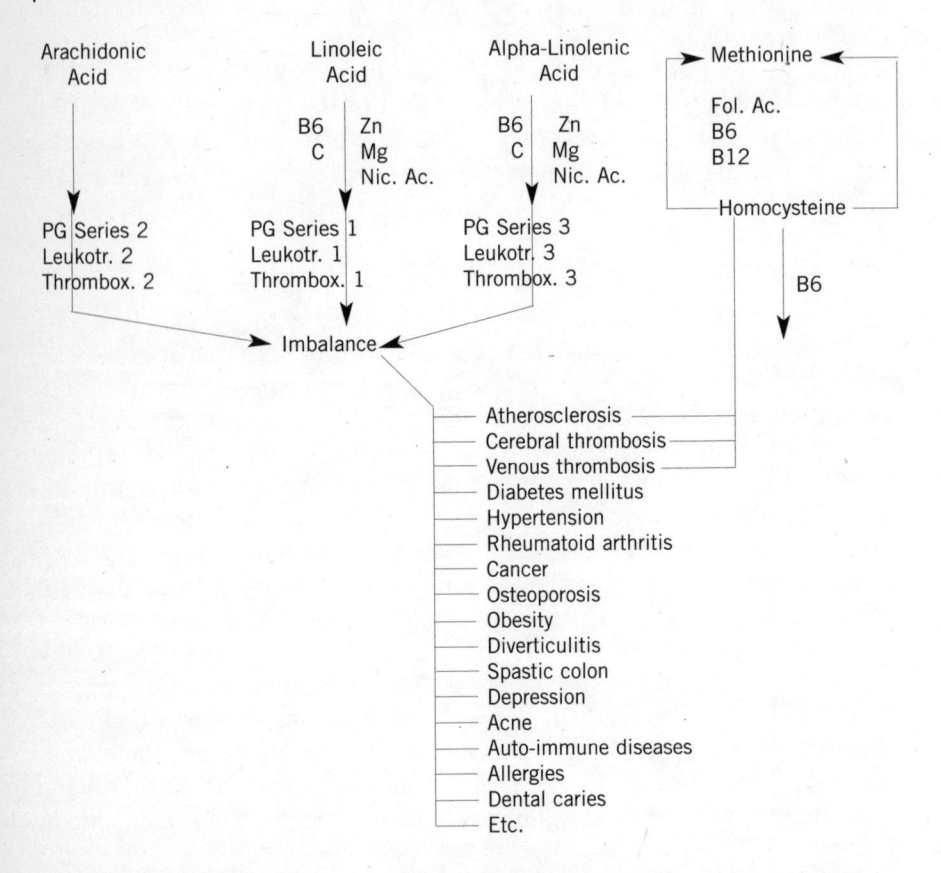

```
Arachidonic        Linoleic        Alpha-Linolenic      Methionine
   Acid              Acid               Acid
                                                        Fol. Ac.
                  B6    Zn          B6    Zn            B6
                  C     Mg          C     Mg            B12
                        Nic. Ac.          Nic. Ac.
                                                        Homocysteine
PG Series 2      PG Series 1       PG Series 3
Leukotr. 2       Leukotr. 1        Leukotr. 3
Thrombox. 2      Thrombox. 1       Thrombox. 3                 B6

                        Imbalance

                        Atherosclerosis
                        Cerebral thrombosis
                        Venous thrombosis
                        Diabetes mellitus
                        Hypertension
                        Rheumatoid arthritis
                        Cancer
                        Osteoporosis
                        Obesity
                        Diverticulitis
                        Spastic colon
                        Depression
                        Acne
                        Auto-immune diseases
                        Allergies
                        Dental caries
                        Etc.
```

Fig 8.1. The probable origin of the greater majority of Western diseases. Note the key role of micronutrients in balancing and controlling fatty acids, prostaglandins, leukotrienes, thromboxanes and homocysteine.

Hypertension (HT) or High Blood Pressure (HBP)

In measuring blood pressure (BP) a rubber cuff of required width (wider in arms of increased mass) is placed around the upper arm. With the aid of a hand (or electronically controlled) pressure bulb, air is pumped into the rubber cuff, and with the aid of a stethoscope on an artery below the cuff, BP is measured on a sphygmomanometer. The upper systolic pressure is when the pulse beat becomes audible as the pressure in the manometer drops, and the diastolic pressure is when the pulse beat disappears. This BP should only be determined by an experienced doctor or nurse.

The normal BP is approximately 120/80, measured in millimetres mercury. There is considerable controversy as to when the BP should be considered high. The diastolic pressure is considered a better indication of HBP than the systolic. HBP should only be considered to be present if the BP is found to be high on three separate occasions with reasonable intervals of hours or even days. Frequently the first meeting with a doctor in a white coat, pumping up a cuff on the patient's arm, is enough to push up the BP, known as "white coat HBP".

In a small percentage of cases, 5-10%, HBP can be caused by a kidney or endocrine condition. The majority of these cases can be cured by medication or surgery. For the rest, 90-95%, the cause has for a very long time been unknown. Convention has it that if the cause of a common disease is unknown, it is called **essential**. Consequently the far greater majority of HBP cases are known as essential hypertension. However, there is every reason to believe that the cause of HBP is now becoming known.

Convention has it that a **normal** BP is defined as below 140/85, age disregarded.

A **mildly high** BP has a diastolic pressure of between 90 and 104, and individualisation of treatment has been conventionally recommended.

The following values indicate **serious** HBP according to the World Health Organisation.

Persons:	
younger than 20 years:	130/85 mm Hg;
20-29 years:	160/95 mm Hg;
30-64 years:	170/95 mm Hg;
65 years and older:	175/95 mm Hg.

It is important to note that it is universally recognised that although effective antihypertensive therapy with conventional drugs reduces the risk of stroke, it has little impact, if any, on lowering the incidence of heart attacks (World Congress on Risk Factor Management in Heart Disease, Copenhagen, Sept. 15, 1990).

Original Description. It is difficult to determine whether HBP was present before food refinement in 1880, since the inflatable rubber cuff sphygmomanometer was developed only in 1896 by an Italian, Riva-Rocci. The term **essential hypertension** was introduced by Theodore Janeway in 1904, using it to mean only a permanent elevation of BP.

Incidence. It is estimated that between 15% and 20% of people living in industrialised countries suffer from HBP, which makes it one of the most prevalent diseases in the world. In the USA a definite difference in incidence between black and white Americans is noted, it being 33% higher in blacks. Yet in traditional tribal communities, no cases of HBP are found, as was noted years ago in studies of the Pygmies of the Congo, Zulus in South Africa, Kung Bushmen in Northern Botswana, New Guinea Highlanders, South American Indians, Pacific Islanders and Australian Aborigines (*Lancet* 1995; 346: 392).

It can therefore be concluded that the greater the industrialisation of a society, the higher the prevalence of HBP. As in atherosclerosis, little doubt exists that HBP has increased considerably since the beginning of the twentieth century. The Framingham study after 36 years estimates that 25% of adults in the USA have hypertension, and that in 78% of the men and in 65% of the women this is due to obesity (*NEJM* 1996; 334: 1571-6).

Prostaglandins. Of all metabolic diseases, hypertension appears to be one of the most susceptible to prostaglandin imbalance. Strong evidence exists which indicates that a deficiency in prostaglandin formation, particularly PGE1, is the primary cause of essential hypertension. In a study, this decrease in PGE1 was the only finding that was present in all cases with essential hypertension (Papanikolaou N., "Hypertension", in *Prostaglandins*, Curtis-Prior P.B., Editor, 1988). PGE1 has wide functions, including several which normalise heart and blood vessel function, such as blood vessel pressures, inhibit the BP-increasing noradrenaline, increasing blood flow through the kidneys, inhibit certain reactions (lysosome activation) which could lead to heart disease, inhibit thrombosis and inhibit cholesterol formation.

Genetics. It became clear that genetics play a role in HBP when it was discovered that in the application of one of the commonest and oldest BP-lowering drugs, propanolol, twice the dosage was necessary in black Africans to achieve the same results as in whites, while only half the dosage was necessary in Chinese to achieve the same results (*Lancet*, Editorial, 2 March 1989). Possibly polymorphism or different adaptions of an active enzyme, dibrosoquinone hydroxylase, plays a role. A few more important findings are that renin, the hormone controlling blood flow through the kidney, is higher in whites than in blacks, while another hormone, aldosterone, controlling blood pressure through its effect on sodium is also in higher concentration in urine of whites than in blacks. Furthermore it has been established that potassium intake in the diet is lower in blacks than in whites.

These differences are undoubtedly due to genetic variations over thousands of years, occasioned by changes in climate and the availability of water and salts, including potassium, in the diets near or away from the warmer equatorial areas. Some researchers have suggested that skin colour, due to its effect on water metabolism, may play a role in the differences of HBP in races (*JAMA*, Editorial, 6 Feb. 1991).

Conventional treatment of HBP. Of all fields of therapeutics the treatment of HBP has gone overboard in the proliferating manufacture of drugs. Competition is rife, with claims that each new drug on the market is so much more effective than any other, but profitability is the secret criterion. Five groups of drugs are available: the diuretics to lower a high fluid content in the body, as with overweight the adrenergic inhibitors acting on adrenaline and its relatives to lessen the heart pump output; angiotension-converting enzyme inhibitors which lower blood vessel tension in the tissues fed by the heart; the calcium channel blockers which have a similar effect as the former only on other sites; and the direct blood vessel dilators. Many schemes for antihypertensive drug therapy have been proposed, and frequently individual experience shows the way. Most drugs have unpleasant side effects which include heart failure, irregular heartbeat, cold extremities, high blood sugar, low blood potassium, headaches, flushing, constipation, rashes, kidney disturbances, increases in blood cholesterol and triglycerides and an irritating dry cough. Hypertension has, since the increase in heart attack deaths, always been considered as one of the main risk factors in atherosclerosis. Yet, as previously mentioned in this book, the lowering of BP by the conventional drugs has not led to a decrease in deaths from heart attacks. In a controlled study in Seattle it was shown that the use of short-acting calcium channel blockers, especially in high doses, was associated with a 60% increased risk of heart attacks (*JAMA* 1995; 274: 620-25).

Micronutrient genetic treatment. If, as in the case of atherosclerosis, essential hypertension has developed as a result of micronutrient depletion, in whichever genetic race, then micronutrient replacement accompanied by a genetic diet should go so far as to cure essential hypertension. This would indicate that micronutrients should effectively replace all the functions of the above-mentioned hypertensive-treating drugs. There is every reason to believe that they do just that. The biggest losses in the refinement of food are phosphate and magnesium (See Table 2.3). Magnesium has now been shown to have at least two very important functions regarding the heart and hypertension. It acts as an antiarhythmic agent and as a calcium antagonist (*Brit Heart J.*, Editorial, 1992; 68: 441-2). This editorial has suggested that magnesium medication should be the primary therapy in an early diagnosis of HBP. The author has had considerable success in treating Africans and whites with high micronutrient genetic diets, plus micronutrient supplementation with magnesium content of approximately 150 mg per day. Only one single patient did not respond. However, this lady did not respond to any other conventional treatments either, despite extensive referrals to physicians. The African diet included sorghum in its most unrefined form. None of the patients presented with any unpleasant side effects – on the contrary, they commented on their sense of wellbeing and increased energy. The only additional drugs occasionally found to be necessary were diuretics for a temporary period.

Other Nonpharmacological Treatment. Weight reduction in the obese is important. There should be at least a modest decrease in salt intake. A reduction in alcohol intake could be helpful. Physical activity should be stepped up. Avoid stress and apply relaxation as previously described, and if necessary pharmacological treatment may have to be applied for the latter.

Conclusion: It is highly probable that essential HBP was absent or extremely rare before the advent of food processing. Logically a return to the genetic diet of races prior to 1880 should cause a return to normal BP. Due to the unavailability of these diets in modern food manufacturing, a permanent supplement of micronutrients, as mentioned above, is imperative. In the author's experience, the return to normal BP occurred, in the vast majority of cases, within a relatively short period of four to eight weeks. Persons who did not respond favourably to this treatment were grossly overweight.

Diabetes Mellitus Type II (DMII)

Although diabetes (sugar in the urine) was known to Hippocrates (460-370 A.D.), the condition was only named diabetes mellitus by a Greek doctor, Pretaeus (81-138 A.D.).

The incidence of this disease has shown an incredible escalation in the last 100 years. In the USA it increased from 1.2 million cases in 1950 to 5 million in 1975, an increase of more than 300%, while the population only increased by 50% (Barcley J. and Harvey A.M., *Two Centuries of American Medicine*, 1976). Between 1980 and 1987 the number increased from 5.8 million to 6.8 million. A definite difference was noted in genetic races and sexes: white male sufferers increased by 38%; white females remained unchanged; black males increased by 16% and black females by 24%. In 1987 the prevalence in black females was more than twice that in white females, and the prevalence in black males was one-third higher than in white males (*JAMA*, 26 Dec. 1990).

Insulin Dependent Diabetes Mellitus (IDDM or DMI). This type of DM is not considered a modern or Western disease, as it was already known in Hippocrates' time.

As the name denotes, insulin injections under the skin are absolutely necessary to control the condition. Unfortunately, insulin cannot be given by mouth as it is destroyed by the gastric juices. Though many theories have been suggested as to the cause of IDDM, it is now becoming clear that it stems from an auto-immune (or self-directed) attack on the pancreas cells that form insulin. A certain active antibody cell, the helper T-lymphocyte, which is produced in the bone marrow but matures in the immune-controlling thymus, appears to have central command of the whole attack on the insulin-producing beta-cell in the pancreas. The whole action is largely associated (42%) with the genetic region on chromosome 6, the so-called major histocompatibility complex (MCH) or human lymphocytic antigen (HLA), while four other genes play a minor role.

IDDM has one of the strongest associations with HLA genetics so far discovered. Of all IDDM patients, 95% have a HLA DR3 or DR4 association, which can be biochemically determined in any pathology laboratory.

In practice, an individual who is genetically predisposed to IDDM (HLA DR3 or HLA DR4) is exposed to a foreign protein that closely resembles a part of the beta-cell of the pancreas responsible for insulin production. This causes a reaction by other immune-defensive cells (macrophages), unleashing a vigorous immune and destructive response to the foreign protein. Initially the beta-cells can withstand the assault, but eventually they succumb. When about 80% of the cells are destroyed, the symptoms of IDDM develop (high blood sugar, sugar in the urine). Evidence exists that certain bacterial heat-shock proteins may be among the offending foreign proteins stimulating the immune reaction. Frequently an acute virus infection, such as measles, may precipitate the condition.

To repeat, this is not a modern Western disease but is detailed here for the sake of completeness. At present IDDM comprises less than 5% of all diabetics.

The Commoner Diabetes. Because of its late onset in age and insulin not usually needed as treatment, this form is also known as noninsulin dependent diabetes mellitus (NIDDM) or late-onset DM. This form of DM is simply and purely a disease of incorrect diet, especially of refined foods. Approximately 50% of these cases are overweight. Nearly every case has a history of overeating sweetened and refined foods and drinks, such as white bread, cakes, sugared tea and coffee, sweetened beverages, etc. The overworked beta-cells in the pancreas cannot keep up with the onslaught from glucose-laden foods. Finally in middle age or later, the insulin-secreting beta-cells become exhausted and NIDDM occurs. However, not all cases necessarily have a high glucose intake history, but they do have a high refined food intake.

As both IDDM and NIDDM persist, blood vessels become damaged, leading to heart disease, blindness, kidney failure and nerve damage. Even the blood cholesterol is increased. However, heart disease and the increased cholesterol is probably due per se to the unrefined diet and not to diabetes itself.

Here, too, an imbalance of prostaglandins has been shown to play a role, PGE1 once more being central to the pathology (Curtis-Prior, 1988).

South Asian races (Indians, Pakistanis, Sri Lankans, Burmese, Thai, Malaysians, etc.) have an important relationship with NIDDM. Shortly after emigrating to other countries (Britain, Trinidad, South Africa) they develop three diseases, NIDDM, coronary heart disease and high blood pressure, in incidences much higher than found in the local inhabitants (Beckles, G.L.A. et al., *Lancet*, 1986; *BMJ* 1995; 311: 1035-6). Yet back in South Asia the incidences of these diseases are low. McKeigh, P.M. et al. (*Lancet*, 16 Feb. 1991) and others, have suggested an "insulin resistance syndrome", for want of a name. Other minority groups in the USA (blacks, Hispanics and native Americans) develop the same diseases at higher incidences than the general local population. This phenomenon can be explained totally on the basis of different genetic diets as discussed previously.

Conventional treatment. Oral insulin-lowering drugs are available, but all textbooks are unanimous in the opinion that this is no replacement for the correct diet. Frequently by the time that DM (NIDDM) has been discovered in elderly persons it may be fairly advanced in symptoms and pathology with the consequence that oral treatment is urgent. The application of a strict diet, if adhered to conscientiously, could eliminate the use of the drugs within a reasonably short time. If, however, no attention is given to the diet, the chances are good that the disease will progress, and may even eventually necessitate the use of insulin. Once permanent damage to the kidney capillaries has occurred the prognosis is extremely poor. This also applies to the blood vessels of the legs, with the danger of gangrene setting in and necessitating amputations.

Diet. Up to 1983 the recommended diet for DM of all types was a low-carbohydrate, low-fat and high-protein diet. It concentrated particularly on a low sugar intake. However, the serious heart and blood vessel complications, frequently the final killer, did not improve. In 1983 a change of thinking took place, initiated by the British Diabetic Association. They proposed an unrefined carbohydrate diet, which was in fact the genetic micronutrient diet. Its main aim was to lessen the danger of blood vessel and coronary heart disease. Prof Jim Mann of Oxford, in an editorial in the *Journal of the American College of Nutrition* states, "Although these dietary recommendations are directed towards the diabetic populations, they are essentially similar to those recommended by most authorities for the population as a whole." Surely this is enough evidence to suggest that DM II is due to the refinement and other deleterious food manufacturing processes of the last century.

The genetic micronutrient diet is to be applied to both forms of diabetes. In IDDM, which must still be considered incurable, the dosage of insulin required is frequently lowered. In NIDDM, if neither too far advanced nor neglected, there is a real possibility of cure by a strict diet with micronutrients supplementation. Oral insulin-lowering drugs should be decreased gradually as the blood and urinary sugars normalise.

Based on the genetic dietary factors it would appear logical that South Asians who have emigrated to Western countries, as well as other non-Western groups living in Western countries, should, as far as possible, revert to their genetic diets. It is the author's experience that these South Asians do not generally adopt the higher fat diets of their new Western neighbours, but remain on rice as their staple diet. The type of rice now commonly available to the migrant, however, is the refined white rice largely denuded of its micronutrients. A return to the more unrefined brown rice should have a highly beneficial effect on the immigrant's DM, high blood pressure and coronary heart disease.

Rheumatoid Arthritis (RA)

This is one of the most painful and degenerative diseases that can afflict man, causing extremely painful joints. The term **rheumatism** was first coined by De Baillou (1538-1616). The first reasonably accurate description of RA was in 1800 by Landre-Beauvois, but it was Sir Alfred Garrod, a famous British physician, who gave RA its name in 1859.

Gold therapy, introduced in 1929, caused a sensation, but its effect was never substantial, and certainly not worth the cost. Dr Philip Hench made a curious observation that his patients with RA underwent a remission (a temporary improvement) when they developed jaundice or acute liver infection, or when they became pregnant. Wondering what the cause could be, he correctly concluded that an increase of corticosteroids (hormones formed in the supra-renal or sex glands) was the reason. The sick liver was unable to detoxify the steroids normally, while pregnancy normally increased the steroids. This led to treating RA with steroids, with highly satisfactory results. In 1950 Philip Hench and two other scientists, E.C. Kendall and R. Reichstein, were awarded the Nobel Prize for their combined research on steroids.

Immediately after World War II steroids were extensively used for RA, with remarkably good effects – as long as the treatment was continued. When treatment was terminated or even decreased, however, the symptoms would soon return in an aggravated form, worse than before the treatment. Consequently this "wonder drug" soon lost its appeal, particularly as it simultaneously decreased the natural immune reaction. Dangerous side effects and complications also developed, such as gastric ulcers and haemorrhages. Nowadays steroids are still used, but at optimally low levels and rapidly declining dosages so as to avoid affecting the immune system.

Rheumatoid arthritis was probably a rare disease for centuries, but all modern textbooks unanimously confirm that during this last century, the disease has increased considerably. Today approximately 1% of the Western population suffer from it.

The following criteria are applied for the diagnosis of RA:

Morning stiffness in and around joints lasting for at least one hour before maximal improvement is noted.

Swellings of the soft tissues in three or more joints.

Swelling of the proximal (nearest) finger, palm or wrist joints.

The joints are symmetrically affected.

Small nodules (hard swellings) under the skin.

A positive blood test for rheumatoid factor.

Radiographic evidence of erosions or thinning of the bone in hand or wrist joints.

If the first four symptoms have been present for six or more weeks the diagnosis is considered confirmed.

Although the cause of the disease is not known for certain, it appears probable that it is due to a single virus or several viruses that generate an immune reaction, which cross-reacts with its own host tissues, i.e. an autoimmune reaction (Harris E.D., *NEJM*, 3 May 1990).

Genetics. Of all the Western metabolic diseases, RA has probably the most definite genetic background. The susceptibility to developing RA is strongly determined by factors known as receptors on cells belonging to certain major histocompatibility complexes. These are the human lymphocytic antigens known as HLA DR4 or HLA DR1. Blood tests are available to determine the presence of these antigens. Another immune substance, rheumatoid factor, is present in the blood of 70-80% of patients with RA.

Other factors which have been known to play a prominent role in RA are the heat-shock proteins, as certain bacteria and possibly viruses can supress them, thereby aggravating the condition.

Prostaglandins. These, too, have been known to play a prominent role in RA, particularly PGE2 and PGF1 stimulating the lesions, while PGE1 and PGF2 suppress the condition. Again the important PGE1 has a beneficial effect.

Conventional treatment. This is expensive and not very effective, frequently leading to advanced degeneration of the joints which then require curative surgery. Early in the disease a measure of success is obtained with aspirin and corticosteroids. However, corrective prostaglandins, stimulated by micronutrients, have the same effect, but without the unpleasant side effects of gastritis, liver and lung toxicity, and suppression of the natural immune system. Should this conventional treatment be terminated at any stage, the symptoms of RA return in an exaggerated form, something which cannot happen on the permanent genetic micronutrient diet.

Diet. Diet has in the past always been a basic part of the treatment in addition to physiotherapy, temperature regulation, occupational therapy and drugs, but has not had the full recognition it deserves. As RA has increased so extensively with food refinement, it is obvious that a return to the genetic micronutrient diet must lead to improvement. This diet restores the prostaglandin balance (which is what steroids and aspirins attempt to do), restores the immune system (which has obviously been lost), and stimulates the tissue and joint metabolism, thereby restoring normal tissues.

The full diet, concentrating especially on green leafy vegetables, is highly important. Popular books, describing a "Seven Day Cure for RA", based on a high vegetable and fruit diet, may sound somewhat overoptimistic, but have good scientific evidence for success. However, do not forget the rest of the diet.

Experience has taught the author that RA is perhaps the only Western disease in which micronutrient diet and supplementation are not sufficient for acceptable results, and other drugs such as nonsteroidal anti-inflammatory agents will have to be added. However, the latter will act more swiftly and at lower dosages than without micronutrients.

Diseases of a Loss of Immunity

Immunity is the tendency of the body to protect itself from infective and other diseases through the action of antibodies. Sometimes these antibodies react to stimuli that the body would not normally react against, and then auto-immune diseases develop, with disastrous long-term effects.

Normally the body's immunity is in a balanced state, with a number of factors playing a role. The organs controlling immunity are the spleen, the lymphatic vessels, the lymph glands, the bone marrow, and the most important of all, a gland known as the **thymus**. But in fact, all the cells in the body have a built-in mechanism defending the body against bacteria, protozoa, viruses and other undesirable stimuli, via an ever-present immune system.

The central regulating mechanism is undoubtedly situated in the thymus, a small flat organ behind the breastbone just above the heart. Weighing between 10 and 30 g, it significantly contains an old friend PGE1, in its highest concentration in the body, without the presence of any other prostaglandins at all (*Med Hypothesis* 1979; 5: 969-85). PGE1 is therefore an extremely important factor in regulating immunity. But here, too, programming plays a role, for the above-mentioned article indicates that should too much PGE1 be present, it will lower immunity regulation. PGE1's precursor is linoleic acid, the most common polyunsaturated fatty acid in the body. So be warned, excessive PUFAs, as recommended in the AHA's diet, is potentially harmful to the immune system.

Fig 8.2 illustrates the role of micronutrients and PGE1 in controlling the immune system. It is clear that insufficient micronutrients as well as excessive PUFAs are equally harmful, as both mechanisms lower immunity. The unhealthy role of a too high intake of PUFAs was fully discussed in Chapter 3.

Classification of diseases of immunity. Infective diseases such as bronchitis, pneumonia, meningitis, otitis, tonsillitis, etc. are all diseases which are treated by antibiotics, and which the human body fights with its own natural antibodies and anti-infective agents. It is clear that the human immune system is a delicately balanced structure, a veritable computer, built up by the experience of thousands of years of battle against infective diseases. However, the immune system not only battles infective diseases but also other metabolic diseases. Up to the end of the nineteenth century the defence against the latter appeared to be reasonably effective.

Since this century, however, this defence has become less effective and a new group – or a considerable increase of previously rare – diseases have developed. The immunity mechanism itself has become a disease. These diseases can be classified into the following groups.

THE OTHER GREATER METABOLIC DISEASES • 145

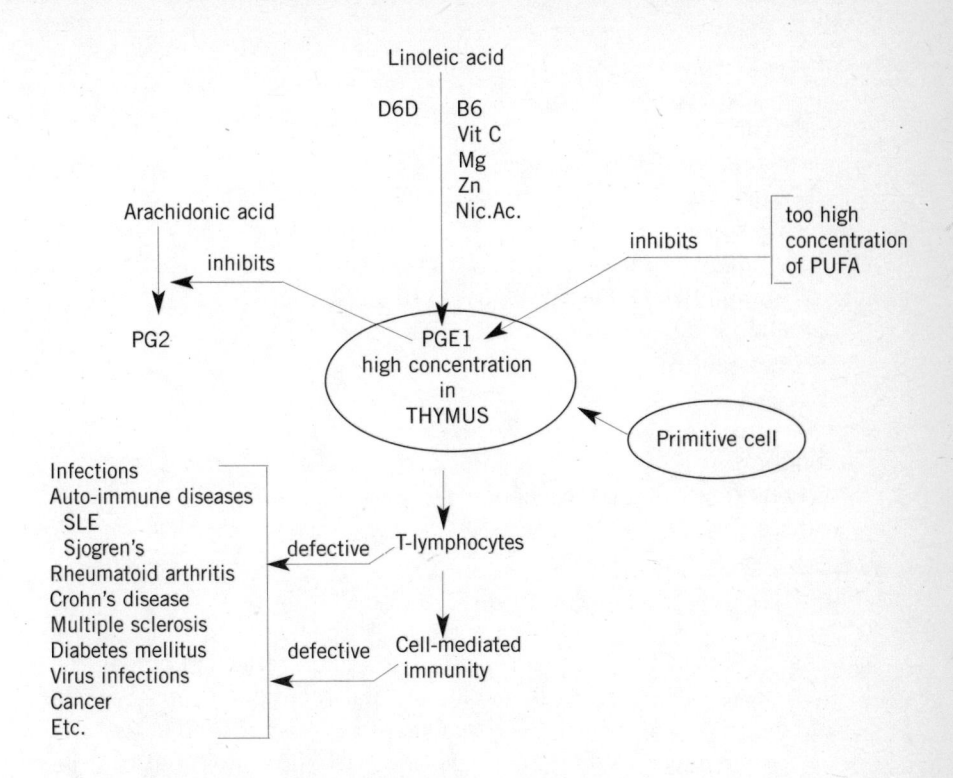

```
                        Linoleic acid
                                │
                    D6D │  B6
                        │  Vit C
                        │  Mg
                        │  Zn                             ┌ too high
   Arachidonic acid     │  Nic.Ac.         inhibits       │ concentration
           │            │                                 │ of PUFA
           │  inhibits  ▼                ▼
           ▼         ╭─────────────╮
          PG2        │    PGE1     │
                     │high concentration│
                     │     in      │◄──── Primitive cell
                     │   THYMUS    │
                     ╰─────────────╯
                            │
  Infections                ▼
  Auto-immune diseases
    SLE          defective   T-lymphocytes
    Sjogren's   ◄─────────       │
  Rheumatoid arthritis            ▼
  Crohn's disease      defective  Cell-mediated
  Multiple sclerosis  ◄─────────  immunity
  Diabetes mellitus
  Virus infections
  Cancer
  Etc.
```

SLE = Systemic lupus erythematosis; D6D = Delta-6-desaturase.

Fig 8.2. The control of immunity and immune-related diseases by prostaglandins and micronutrients. Note particularly the balanced role of PUFA's.

    Allergies:
      hayfever (rhinitis)
      asthma
      eczema (atopic dermatitis)
      heat bumps (urticaria)
      red eyes (conjunctivitis)
      mid-ear infections (otitis media)
      milk allergies (this may be due to genetic differences of lactase)
      wheat allergies (gluten)
    Auto-Immune Diseases:
      systemic lupus erythematosis (SLE)
      Sjogren's disease
      scleroderma

multiple sclerosis
Addison's disease of the thyroid
spastic colon
hyperthyroidism (Grave's disease)
Crohn's disease
pernicious anaemia
primary biliary cirrhosis
Loss of Immunity as a Partial Aspect of the Disease:
rheumatoid arthritis
diabetes mellitus
cancer
acne
myelofibrosis
infections (bacterial, protozoal, viruses)
  in the elderly
Primary Loss of Immunity:
Aids

Asthma. As asthma is the most common and serious condition among the acute immune diseases, it must receive special mention. It has become twice as common in the past 20 years in most Western countries, and change in diet is more likely than air pollution or house-dust mites to be the cause (*Thorax* 1994; 49: 171-4; *Thorax* 1996; 51: 59-63). There is also growing evidence that prolonged use of inhaled steroids, as is frequently applied, reduces the thickness of bone (*J Royal Coll Physic*, London 1996; 30: 128-32).

Systemic lupus erythematosis (SLE). This, the commonest of the auto-immune diseases, also has a genetic distribution, the rate being higher in Afro-Caribbeans (207/100 000) and in Asians (50/100 000) than in whites (20/100 000 (*Annals of Rheum Dis* 1994; 53: 675-80). Data from nearly 70 000 women in the Nurses' Health Study suggest that those using postmenopausal oestrogen treatment doubled their risk of developing SLE (*Ann Int Med* 1995; 122: 430-3).

The role of micronutrients in immunity. Vitamins, only discovered at the turn of the 19th century, were very soon recognised as playing a key role in the maintenance of good health and in the body's ability to resist disease. Unfortunately, and as could be expected, when antibiotics were discovered, the medical profession immediately started relying exclusively on their new-found wonder treatment and forgot about the beneficial effects of vitamins. However, one doctor, Abe Axelrod, continued experiments in which he applied vitamins to diseases, with highly satisfactory results.

But the antibiotic era is waning thanks to numerous antibiotics losing the battle against resistant bacteria. In 1994 over 100 antibiotics were currently approved in the USA (*Science* 1994; 264: 362-3). The cost of developing a new nonbacterial resistant antibiotic is now so exhorbitant that it may become too expensive for use. Consequently the medical profession is forced to return to micronutrients. Already in 1975 a subcommittee of the National Academy of Science in the USA took the topic of malnutrition and the immune system out of the mothballs. By this time, minerals had been recognised as an additional factor in aiding immunity, mainly as co-factors for enzymes.

Between 31 May and 2 June 1989 an International Congress on Micronutrients and Immune Functions was held in New York under the auspices of the New York Academy of Science. In this way significant recognition was afforded the role of micronutrients in this field.

Micronutrient Treatment of Immune Diseases. As it would take much time and space if each disease listed above were individually discussed, the basic principles of micronutrient treatment of all the above diseases will be combined. The genetic micronutrient diet is applicable to all of them.

Initially, conventional treatment with corticosteroids may have to be applied. However, as balancing of the prostaglandins has the same effect as the corticosteroid treatment, only slightly delayed, the latter treatment need to be applied only briefly. Corticosteroid treatment has side effects and a suppression of certain normal natural immune reactions, thereby possibly aggravating herpes simplex (fever blisters), osteoporosis, thrombosis and peptic ulcers. Long-term corticosteroid use can lead to increased blood pressure, increased weight, increased blood sugar and increased blood fats. Micronutrients and the corresponding diet, being natural substances, have none of these side effects.

It has been the author's experience that laboratory investigations of blood immunoglobulins (IgG, IgA, IgM and IgE) are advised. Should any of these investigations be abnormal or near-abnormal (blood values are not a good reflection of tissue values), booster injections of immunoglobulins are necessary, once every three months for a total period of nine months, to hasten a return to normal immunity.

The acute reactions of an allergy, such as an itchy rash, tissue swelling, an asthma attack, uncontrolled sneezing, some of which could lead to sudden death, are due to a release of histamine by reacting cells known as mast cells. The enzyme necessary to metabolise histamine is **histamine methyltransferase.** All methyltransferases require magnesium as a co-factor, and magnesium is the mineral with the highest loss in food manufacturing (68% in bread, 93% in rice, 74% in maize). Magnesium has a moderating effect on the allergic reactions and treatment with it is imperative.

The above prescribed treatment does not necessarily cure all the immunity diseases, but definitely improves the condition and keeps it at bay.

A word on Aids. Aids is not considered a metabolic disease as defined in this book. However, as expected, certain short-term studies with micronutrient treatment have shown a lengthening and improvement of life expectations. Even homocysteine may play a role. Increased concentrations of a reduced form of homocysteine could possibly cause the formation of increased oxygen compounds, leading to accelerated immunity deterioration and increased HIV action (*Am J Clin Nutr* 1996; 63: 242-8).

Cancer

Of all diseases, ancient or modern, cancer is generally the most dreaded of all, due to the anticipation of pain, suffering and debility, not only from the disease itself but also from the treatment. Little doubt exists that the incidence of cancer is increasing. At the same time it is a disease which can be completely alleviated, sometimes even prevented, through a lifetime of simple common-sense action.

In the developed world cancer is the second largest killer disease, responsible for approximately 20% of annual deaths (Cohen L.A., *Scientific American*, Nov. 1987).

Of this, cigarette smoking is responsible for 30% of all cancer deaths, and heavy alcohol consumption for 3% of all cancer deaths.

In a review article (Davis D.E. et al., *Lancet*, 25 Aug. 1990) the trends in different cancer incidences are recorded. In Italy, Japan, Germany, England, Wales and the USA stomach cancer declined, but cancers of the brain, central nervous system, breast, kidney, multiple myeloma, non-Hodgkins lymphoma and melanoma increased over five years. Lung cancer started to decline in men under age 85, women under age 60, and men under age 45 in England, Wales and the USA.

Cancer linked to cigarette smoking, asbestos, and dietary fat was more frequent in the developed world, while cancer linked to food contaminants, preservatives and infectious diseases was more frequent in the developing world. Men in North America and North Europe had 75% less liver cancer and 30 times more lung cancer than men in West and Central Africa. Japanese women emigrants to Hawaii had half the risk of stomach cancer and twice the risk of breast cancer than in locals. In England and Wales stomach, colon and rectum cancers were declining, while lung, pancreas, prostate, ovary and breast cancers were increasing. In the USA since 1950 stomach, rectum, thyroid cancers and Hodgkins disease were declining, while lung, breast, cervix, uterus, and kidney cancers and non-Hodgkins lymphoma were increasing. Important was that environmental determinants affecting cancer mainly on diet were increasing, while improvements in food storage and reduction of preservatives caused a decrease in cancers.

The above all point very strongly to the role of micronutrient dietary loss and incorrect genetic dietary factors as the main cause of cancer.

It is becoming apparent that treatment of cancer with drugs suppressing the immune system, such as in chemotherapy and radiotherapy, leads to an increase in risk of other cancers developing, such as breast cancer under the age of 40 years if the patient, when young, was treated for Hodgkin's lymphoma (*NEJM* 1996; 344: 745-51), and has potentially devastating side effects in damaging the heart (*Heart* 1996; 75: 591-5).

The following findings are quoted from the unanimous opinions in animal experimentation that polyunsaturated fats cause cancer.

Graham S., 1983, *Epidemiological Reviews*: "The recommendation to reduce one's animal fat intake, for example, is based on rather sparse epidemiological data . . . Indeed, the best data on experimentation suggested that PUFAs are more important than animal fats in increasing the risk of cancer."

Carroll K.K., 1984, *JAOCS*: "Dietary PUFAs increased the yield of mammary tumors in rats more effectively than saturated fats."

Stemmermann G.N., 1984, *Cancer Research*: "We found a statistically significant negative association between colon cancer and the intake of saturated fats."

Clement I.P., 1984, *Nutrition and Cancer*: " . . . the effect of selenium in cancer is accentuated only in the presence of unsaturated fat intake."

Reddy B.S., 1985, *Progress in Food and Nutritional Science*: "Diets containing 20% corn oil or 20% safflower oil increased colon tumors in rats as to diets containing 5% corn oil or 5% safflower oil."

Palmer S., 1985, *Progress in Food and Nutritional Science*: "When total fat intake is low PUFAs appear to be more effective than saturated fats in enhancing tumors." (Yet this is exactly what the AHA recommends in its "prudent diet".)

Cohen L.A., 1987, *Scientific American*: "High fat diets rich in certain fatty acids promote the formation of tumors, whereas similar diets high in other fatty acids do not . . . High fat diets in linoleic acids act as promotors; similar diets rich in oleic acid (from olive oil) and fish oils do not act as promotors."

Drug companies, when wishing to place a new drug on the market, must see to it that it undergoes strict animal experimentation tests. Any sign that the product causes cancer automatically disqualifies it. Increased vegetable oils and margarine, the latter especially with its high abnormal transfatty acids and abnormal cisfatty acids, would never have passed the tests.

Dietary Factors Playing a Role in Cancer. A vast amount of research has been carried out in this field. A positive role for dietary factors has been confirmed by recent research (Davis et al., *Lancet*, 1990; Schatzkin A. et al., *JAMA*, 1989. International Congress on Micronutrients and Immune Functions, New York).

The causes can be classified as follows:
1. Highly significant for cancer:
    increased polyunsaturated fats;
    presence of abnormal transfatty acids;
    decreased vitamin A and carotene;
    decreased vitamin E;
    decreased vitamin B6;
    decreased selenium;
    decreased zinc;
    decreased fibre;
    decreased vegetables (of cruciform type);
    decreased fruit;
    increased alcohol intake;
    increased aflotoxins (in grain foods);
    increased nitrates (in vegetables, drinking water, cured meats, cigarette smoke–nitrosamines);
    increased peroxides and oxidants (from heated vegetable oils).
2. Moderately significant for cancer:
    increased total fats;
    decreased vitamin B1 (Thiamin);
    decreased vitamin B2 (Riboflavine);
3. Slightly significant for cancer:
    increased saturated fats;
    increased animal fats;

      increased refined carbohydrates (sugar);
      increased chocolates;
      increased starchy foods;
      decreased copper;
      decreased iodine;
      decreased calcium;
      decreased iron.
4. Highly controversial:
      increased total energy calories;
      decreased or increased blood cholesterol;
      increased protein;
      increased red meat (only selective, e.g. Japanese);
      decreased vitamin C;
      decreased vitamin D (only selective, ? genetic);
      increased coffee.

It has been estimated that approximately 35% of cancers are due to dietary factors. This figure, however, does not take into consideration the recently discovered effect of micronutrients on the immune system (Horrobin D.F., *Med Hypothesis*, 1979). Consequently, dietary factors can be considered as the most important factor in cancer, as high as 65%.

A few forms of cancer require special mention.

Lung Cancer. Between 1950 and 1990 death rates from lung cancer in the USA increased from 13 to 50 per 100 000 (*Mortality and Morbidity Weekly Reports* 1993; 42: 657-66). Lung cancer deaths exceed those from breast cancer in both black and white women, though only a quarter of American women now smoke. Though passive inhalation by nonsmokers may play a role, the probable cause in the majority of cases is dietary faults.

Breast Cancer. This form of cancer is increasing steadily although only about 4% of women in Western communities will develop it (*Science* 1995; 269: 771-3). For nearly 300 years it has been known to have a high rate in nuns, but now the high-risk groups include executives, teachers, administrators and professionals (*Am J Pub Health* 1993; 83: 1311-5). Previous explanations such as late childbearing are not supported in present studies.

A breast cancer susceptibility gene was discovered in 1990, dubbed BRCA1, in the long arm of chromosome 17. Though a positive family history has been suspected for many years as a risk factor in breast cancer, this gene is only present in 5% of cases (*JAMA* 1995; 273: 1702-3). So serious is this gene considered that some authorities advise breast removal at a relatively young age before cancer occurs. It is reasonable to believe that the other main cause is dietary, and a family history is probably purely due to families following the same diets.

Prostate Cancer. This is now being considered the most common cancer among men, especially over the age of 50 years. However, the prognosis is much more favourable than with breast cancer, even if the incidence is nearly 50%. In a study in Connecticut men aged 65 to 75 years with clinically diagnosed cancer had a survival rate not significantly different from that of the general population (*JAMA* 1995; 274: 626-31).

Both prostate cancer and prostate hypertrophy (benign enlargement) can cause an increase in blood prostate-specific antigen (PSA). It is only when a steady increase in PSA takes place that surgical removal may be indicated. The advice is therefore to follow a genetic micronutrient diet with micronutrient supplementation and no surgery.

Lymphatic Leukaemia. The one big bright spot in cancer is that this condition in children is curable in 80% of cases (*NEJM* 1994; 329: 1289-93).

Micronutrient Treatment. The full genetic micronutrient diet should be vigorously applied. Particular attention should be given to yellow and dark green leafy vegetables (spinach, squash, broccoli, cabbage), carrots, brown rice, pumpkin, asparagus, tomatoes, cantaloupes, apricots, pawpaws, and peaches. Egg yolks, full-cream milk, nuts and germ oil are important (and forget about the cholesterol content). One medical doctor in the USA practically cured himself of widespread prostatic cancer on a diet of basically brown rice (Sattilaro A.J., *Recalled for Life*, Avon Press, 1982). Add to the above the basic foodstuffs of whole-wheat bread and unrefined cereals, as well as wheat germ (or germ oil). In this way a high natural micronutrient intake is obtained, as well as the antioxidants vitamin E, vitamin A and beta-carotene. Multimicronutrient supplementation is absolutely necessary.

If cancer is already present, supplementation in the form of a multimicronutrient tablet or liquid should be added daily. Only normal cells will be stimulated by this supplementation, thereby suppressing the development of the cancer cells, and improving the patients' general condition and ability to fight cancer via the immune system (Sinclair H.M., *Human Nutr*, 1984). Even during chemotherapy the addition of the above diet and micronutrient supplementation has the effect of lessening the unpleasant side effects of chemotherapy, such as hair loss, nausea and weakness.

Depression

Depression is considered by many as a stigma, but if we look at the list of known sufferers this is undoubtedly incorrect. It may even be a sign of greater things. These sufferers include, many by their own admission, Winston Churchill, Billy Graham, Hans Christian Anderson, Barbra Streisand, Carol Burnett, Billie-Jean King, Peter Sellers, John F. Kennedy, Arthur Conan Doyle, even Sigmund Freud, Victor Hugo, Thomas Edison, Charles Dickens, Samuel Johnson, W.B. Yeats, Abraham Lincoln and Mark Twain. So if you are a "sufferer" you are in very good company.

In an article in the *British Journal of General Practice* 1996; 46: 207-8, it is estimated that as many as 95% of patients in general practice suffer from depression in some way or another. The teachings of Sigmund Freud (1856-1939), in which so much importance was placed on the instincts of sex and aggression, are now no longer accepted. In Dr Willis's *Case Book*, in which a number of cases are described suggesting depression (1650-1652), nearly all could be considered nearer hypochondriac. However, little doubt exists that depression and other psychiatric disorders have increased considerably in the past century.

One could possibly believe that an increased number of external factors cause depression, such as being bombarded by bad news through the media, work and mental stress, financial problems and complicated interrelationships of different sorts. Though these undoubtedly play a role, it is becoming abundantly clear that psychochemistry (the effect of body chemical substances on the mood) is of fundamental importance.

These biochemical compounds are highly concentrated in the brain, their function being to transmit nerve impulses to the necessary parts of the brain thus the name neurotransmitters. As in the rest of the body, enzymes and their vitamin and mineral co-factors play an important regulating role. Here too, enzyme polymorphism causes different problems in different individuals. The most active of these neurotransmitters are dopamine, norepinephrine (or noradrenaline), the forerunner of epinephrine (or adrenaline), and serotonin. Other regulating neurotransmitters are acetylcholine (carrying impulses into muscles), and gamma-amino-butyrate (GABA, probably playing a regulatory role in epilepsy) (Wells K.B. et al., *JAMA*, Aug. 1989).

Fig 8.3 illustrates the effects of five neurotransmitters on a person's moods. Note particularly the role of the micronutrients folate, iron, vitamin B6, vitamin C, magnesium and calcium. Should a shortage of micronutrients be present, as there most decidedly is in a Western diet,

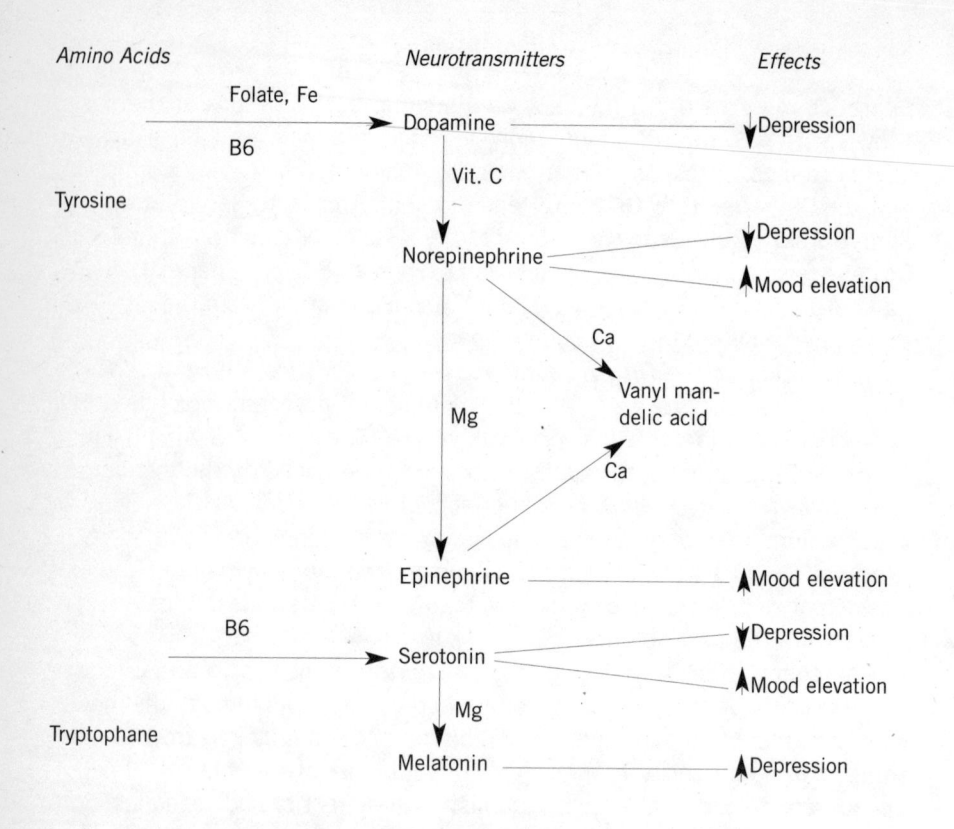

```
Amino Acids            Neurotransmitters              Effects

              Folate, Fe
              ─────────────►  Dopamine ───────────────  ▼ Depression
              B6
Tyrosine
                              │ Vit. C
                              ▼
                              Norepinephrine ─────────  ▼ Depression
                                                        ▲ Mood elevation
                                        ╲ Ca
                                         ╲
                                          ▼
                                     Vanyl man-
                              Mg      delic acid
                                          ▲
                                         ╱
                                        ╱ Ca
                              ▼
                              Epinephrine ─────────────  ▲ Mood elevation

              B6
              ─────────────►  Serotonin ──────────────  ▼ Depression
                                                        ▲ Mood elevation
                              │ Mg
                              ▼
Tryptophane                   Melatonin ───────────────  ▲ Depression
```

▼ decreased concentration; ▲ increased concentration

Fig 8.3. The effects of neurotransmitters, formed from two amino acids, on mood. Note particularly the importance of micronutrients (folate, iron, vitamin B6, magnesium and calcium) in the normal metabolism of neurotransmitters.

mood changes, particularly depression, can become very common. Some persons may react more than others to this micronutrient loss, indicating a sensitivity due to enzyme polymorphism.

Conventional treatment has been by means of antidepressant drugs, all in some manner stimulating the neurotransmitters or their receptors to normalise function. However, the side effects of these drugs are extremely unpleasant – a dry mouth, dizziness, drowsiness, agitation, blurred vision, excessive sweating, muscle tremors and interference with sexual function. Yet all this could be avoided with high concentrations of micronutrients, either as a supplementation and/or in the genetic diet.

Magnesium alone has a calming and sedative effect, due to its function as depicted in Fig 8.3, and can be administered at night ensuring a good night's rest.

With the majority of conventional treatments satisfactory results are usually only seen after three weeks, whereas with micronutrients results are obtained much sooner. With severe depression conventional treatment may still be necessary, but usually only for a short while.

It is interesting to note that the cost of developing new psychotropic drugs in the early 1970s in the USA was $121 million, but by the early 1980s this had risen to $279 million (*Psychopharmacology: the Fourth Generation of Progress*, New York, Raven Press, 1995).

CHAPTER 9

A DIET FOR OVERWEIGHT

Obesity is really widespread.
JOSEPH O. KERN II

Overmass and Obesity

Everybody jokes about being too fat, if not personally, then about others. Denis Norden of *My Word* fame said, "There was only one occasion in my life when I put myself on a strict diet and I can tell you, hand on heart, it was the most miserable afternoon I have ever spent." However, to many it is a serious problem, be it imaginary or not. It can obstruct romance, destroy marriage, and shorten life.

Overmass and obesity differ slightly by definition. With the aid of a tape measure and scale this difference can be measured at home, through the **body mass index** (BMI).

$$BMI = \frac{\text{Bodymass in Kg}}{\text{Height in metres}^2} = \frac{M}{H^2}$$

A BMI below 24 for females or below 25 for males is considered as not being overmass.

A BMI between 24 and 27 for females and between 25 and 27 for males is considered as overmass.

A BMI over 27 for both sexes is considered as obesity.

Denis Burkitt in his book, *Don't Forget Fibre in Your Diet*, 1980, states that portraits of kings, queens and courtiers before the beginning of the eighteenth century reveal slim-bodied persons, and very few illustrations from the ancient civilisations of Egypt, Assyria, Rome and Greece depict fat persons. In East Africa in the 1920s Burkitt noted that fat Africans were rare. Twenty years later the picture had changed considerably, and in both Africa and Western communities obesity and overmass had become common.

Overmass and obesity therefore satisfy our definition and criteria for a modern or Western disease. This does not necessarily indicate overeating, although it can be an important factor, but it can also mean eating the wrong food.

The Role of Fibre

Burkitt was one of the earliest researchers to stress the importance of fibre, especially as a mass-lowering factor. Fibre is very important in absorbing fluid and thereby causing an increase in bulk of intestine content, especially of the large bowel. This, in turn, increases the peristaltic action of the bowel, i.e. the rythmic contraction of the bowel's circular muscles, thereby speeding the increased content into the rectum. The result is larger and more frequent stools. In Hippocrates' time (460-370 BC), it was natural to pass two to three stools per day, a far cry from present-day Western constipation.

Fibre's effect is largely a mechanical one. However, natural fibre cannot easily be separated from its associated bran, 44% of the total fibre (see Table 7.2). The nonfibre part of the bran has probably the highest concentration of micronutrients of all foods known. This is why bran has so many advantageous effects on health, some of which have mistakenly been attributed to fibre. Indeed, it is frightening to remember that up until recently bran was considered good only for pigs.

Prostaglandins. The gastro-intestinal system is one of the best studied regarding prostaglandin metabolism (Curtis-Prior, 1988). With the ever-present prostaglandin imbalance prevailing, a wide variety of undesirable effects can develop, such as intestinal fluid abnormalities, less intestinal action, ulcers in the stomach wall, loss of certain liver functions, abnormal acid secretion in the stomach, abnormal stomach wall activity, diarrhoea and limited gall flow from the liver.

The Obesity Gene

It has been clear for many years that obesity and overweight is not only a result of overeating. Obese persons usually have at least one obese parent, and in many cases obesity, or its opposite, slenderness, may skip a generation. If you are looking for a future slender spouse, don't look only at the parents, have a peep at the grandparents too, in person or in a photograph.

The reason for this has recently been discovered, and of course it has to do with genes. The body has a complex, highly sophisticated system for regulating its fat stores (*NEJM* 1995; 332: 673-4, and 679-80). There appears to be a set point for body fat, also called the **adipostat,** in the lower part of the brain, the hypothalamus, where it forms a network. This serves to maintain an internal image of the proper amount of fat tissue for this individual's body. The whole controlling action lies in a gene in chromosome 6, now aptly named the **ob-gene**, but it is highly probable that other genes with lesser action, as is frequently found in genetics, may still be discovered.

The set point compares the actual amount of fat tissue with the internal ideal as genetically determined, and then takes steps to minimise the difference. This occurs through metabolic adjustments in an effort to return the body fat to the baseline level. However, if the micronutrients necessary for the metabolic adjustments are decreased, this mechanism cannot take place.

The general trend during the lifetime of most people is to gain weight, with a few lucky exceptions, and, typically, a 70 kg man acquires about 10 kg of fat in 20 years. These adipostats are consequently reset upward. The adipostat can also be reset by external factors, such as drugs, certain properties of the diet (most certainly micronutrients), and the habitual level of physical activity.

A few practical lessons are to be learnt from the above. Do not expect to develop a model's figure if your parents are porky. Never expect to regain your teenage figure after your thirties or forties. Allow for the middle-age spread; it is inevitable. Watch your teenage daughters and sons if they attempt to have more slender figures than your own teenage figures; they may be heading for anorexia nervosa or bulimia.

Losing Mass for Health Reasons

Mass-losing diets with claims such as "a kilogram lost per day or more", are potentially dangerous and the results short-lived. They may be effective for a few weeks, but after that they become impossible to continue with, affect general health adversely, and a return to the original mass or more is the rule. To be effective, the loss of mass must be gradual and the person will have to be satisfied with one to three kilograms lost per month, until a stable mass has been attained and maintained.

The following modifications and emphases of the genetic micronutrient diet are proposed:

Restrict breakfast foods strictly to unrefined sources, Weet-Bix, Hi-Bulk Bran, All-Bran, mueslis and unrefined mealie meal (maize, straight-run).

Avoid oats. It is not effective enough because it has only been in general West-European use since 1860.

Use natural bran freely – if necessary in fruit drinks, and also a half-hour before meals to suppress appetite.

Use only whole-wheat bread.

Use butter sparingly, and avoid all margarines strictly.

Fruits: give preference to prunes, figs, apples, bananas.
Add moderate milk (skimmed only for excessive mass loss; remember a cholesterol-lowering factor is being lost by doing this), minimal sugar (honey is a good replacement).
Give preference to crisp-bread sandwiches.
Salads: give preference to cabbage, spinach, carrots and tomatoes.
Avoid business lunches, unless you can strictly apply the diet.
Avoid cream, full-fat cheese, ice cream and nondairy creamers.
Use avocado pears sparingly.
Restrict daily cheese to a piece the size not exceeding that of a matchbox.
Red meat and sausages must be strictly lean.
Eat only steamed or boiled fish, no fried fish.
Cook vegetables for a very short time, particularly green beans, brinjals, carrots, cabbages, cauliflower, broccoli, and dry beans.
Rice: Use only brown rice.
Strictly avoid polony, salami, caviar, bone marrow, shrimps, viennas, brains, liver, kidneys.
Avoid alcohol strictly.
Avoid sweets, sugared fruits and unnatural beverages.
Avoid all cake and confectionary.
Avoid smoking.
Take part in active relaxing exercise. Remember, any loss of mass from exercise alone without a diet will only be of very short duration.

The Beauty Queen Diet

This diet is mainly for entrants to beauty competitions, but anyone who seriously wishes to lose weight may follow it. Elizabeth Taylor followed a similar diet when she regained her youthful figure at over 50 years of age. She unfortunately lost it again when her ob-gene eventually took over.

Motivation to lose mass. For any success to be achieved the will to lose mass must be strong and efforts persevered with tenaciously. Take some unusual steps, such as pasting your least flattering photograph on your mirror. Do not undergo a forced starvation shortly before your presentation day, be it a beauty competition or an important date. Do not expect dramatic initial effects, but be satisfied with 1-2 kg mass loss per week. If your motivation fades, seek help from a mass-loss club or institution.

Appetite suppressants. Be careful of dramatic claims. Some act through suppressing seretonin, which could also cause depression. Furthermore mass problems may become more severe after diet cessation. The healthiest and cheapest suppressor is wheat bran, two tablespoons in fruit juice half an hour before meals.

Exercise. Take part in a healthy, vigorous programme. Enjoyable exercise, such as walking, tennis, swimming, is the most profitable, and at the same time the least expensive.

Starvation. Avoid strictly, and do not miss a meal during the day.

High fibre concentrate. This can be liberally used, with or between meals, to suppress appetite. Use, however, only natural digestive bran to avoid impaction of the bowels.

The Diet

Use the **3:2:3 plan**; three items of food for breakfast, two for lunch, and three for the evening meal.

Breakfast
Do not omit. Vary the main item between:
One slice of whole-wheat bread with moderate butter and Marmite, Bovril, Fray Bentos or other natural smears;
One Weet-Bix biscuit, or serving of Hi-Bulk Bran or Muesli, with skimmed milk and minimal sugar or honey;
One poached or boiled egg, mixed with stewed vegetables, or on a toasted slice of whole-wheat bread.

The second item could vary between:
120 ml low-fat yogurt, unsweetened;
half a grapefruit, unsweetened;
stewed prunes and apricot, unsweetened;
one apple;
25 g hazelnuts in yoghurt, unsweetened.

The third item should be one of:
fresh fruit;
juice – tomato, orange, pineapple or any other unsweetened fruit juice (use your imagination);
tea without milk and sugar.

Add wheat bran to control hunger.

Lunch
Do not omit. The first item should be an imaginative soundly-based selection of high-fibre foods with high-micronutrient salads, including some of the following:
sliced spinach, cauliflower, cabbage, (no lettuce);
Brussels sprouts, broccoli;
pineapple, dried apricots;
carrots, peas;
cottage cheese;
tuna, tomatoes, mushrooms;
brazil nuts, almond nuts, cashew nuts;
Do not add mayonnaise.

The second item should be 150 ml portion of orange, apple or pineapple juice (or other unsweetened fruit juice).

Should the pangs of hunger be too much to endure, even after partaking of wheat bran, a single slice of lightly buttered whole-wheat bread, or a single cooked potato (with skin), or a whole-wheat bread roll, lightly buttered, with added Marmite, Oxo or Fray Bentos, can be allowed.

The evening meal
Three items are allowed. The first one is animal protein. The principle of lean red meat four times per week, cooked fish twice per week, and boiled chicken once per week, can be adhered to. The meat must be strictly lean, and all visible fat removed. This item can occasionally be replaced by a seafood salad of shrimps or boiled unrefined spaghetti or macaroni. The latter may be preferred by Mediterraneans.
Consider vegetables as the second item. Give preference to:
cooked brown rice;
steamed cauliflower, broccoli;
fresh peas, asparagus, squashes, baby marrows;
potatoes cooked in their skins;
tomato puree;
onions.

The third item is once more orange, pineapple, apple or other fruit and unsweetened fruit juice.

In-betweens

Wheat bran in fresh fruit juice will control hunger.

Snacks should be restricted to whole-wheat biscuits with vegetable and meat extract smears.

Black sugarless tea is allowed, with artificial sweeteners. An occasional diet cool drink is allowed.

Pure or mineral water is allowed in moderation. Remember, the body contains 60-70% water.

There is no danger attached to the diet as the most important factor, the micronutrient content, is adequate. The big problem is continued motivation. However, once the desired mass is achieved, a return to an adequate and sustained genetic micronutrient diet should be sufficient, aided by an optimum multimicronutrient supplement.

CHAPTER 10

OTHER AND LESSER MODERN DISEASES

It should be the function of medicine to have people die young as late as possible.
ERNEST L. WYNDER

Introduction

Many of the diseases to be discussed in this last chapter are connected to reasonably strong genetic factors. However, we must not be overawed by this fact into believing that little can be done. Genetic factors invariably indicate an **enzyme fault** caused by one major gene plus a few minor genes. Do not confuse this with a dominant genetic disease such as familial hypercholesterolaemia, a far more serious condition.

Furthermore the enzyme faults are never total, and the enzyme can always be stimulated by the correct micronutrients, or even applicable amino acids, so as to apparently and clinically near-normalise the condition, with a seeming disappearance of the disease in many cases. Should the treatment with the necessary genetic diet and micronutrients be discontinued, the disease will return.

Osteoporosis

This is a condition of weakening or thinning of the bone structure due to loss of minerals. Archaeological skeletons have shown that, since ancient times, women have lost bone to a greater extent than men (Armelagos G.J., *Science*, 1969). Up to 50% of people over the age of 65 years from industrialised countries suffer from osteoporosis.

In 1882 Bruns noted that, before the age of 50, hip fractures occurred mainly in men, but after that age were far more common in women. At present hip and wrist fractures are eight to ten times more frequent in women than in men. Fractures of the hip in elderly patients has increased considerably over the past 20 years (Delmi M. et al., *Lancet*, 28 April 1990).

Furthermore, bone fractures, especially of the hip, are less common in blacks, and particularly rare in African blacks (Walker A.R.P., *Lancet*, 5

December 1987). Of hip fractures in Auckland, New Zealand, over a period of 60 years among 1 832 men and 1 774 women, only 16 were Maoris (*NZMJ* 1995; 108: 426-8). It has been shown that blacks have a stronger bone structure than whites.

Two possible mechanisms could explain this difference. One suggests that the thinness of white people's bones is associated with evolutionary changes that helped early humans to make enough vitamin D in their skin when exposed to the lower levels of sunlight nearer the poles, while wearing clothing to protect against the cold (*Ann Rheum Dis* 1996; 55: 335-7).

A more simple and logical explanation is the loss of bone minerals in the genetic diets. Sorghum has been the traditional genetic diet of the black man in Africa. At present the latter has a strong preference for the white super raw maize. This refined grain has 7 times less calcium than the former, 4 times less magnesium, 3 times less phosphate and 5 times less zinc (Table 10.1). Furthermore the white man now also eats a maize containing 3.3 times less calcium, 4 times less magnesium, 3.5 times less phosphate and 4.5 times less zinc.

	WHITE SUPER RAW MAIZE	STRAIGHT-RUN RAW MAIZE	MALTABELLA (SORGHUM) UNCOOKED
	per 100 g		
Fibre (g)	2.6	10.6	1.5
Calcium (mg)	3.0	10.0	21.0
Magnesium (mg)	32.0	123.0	117.0
Phosphate (mg)	71.0	241.0	192.0
Zinc (mg)	0.50	2.30	2.64

Table 10.1. The loss of minerals in maize and sorghum refinement (Ref.: *MRC Food Composition Tables*, 3rd edit., Langenhoven et al., Parow, 1991).

It would appear that the prime candidates for osteoporosis are elderly white women. These persons are, due to institutional and nutritional circumstances, inclined to be underfed. The most effective conventional treatment so far determined for them has been female hormone replacement with oestrogen or oestrogen in combination with progesterone. This hormone treatment has to be delicately balanced, for an excessive dosage could lead to cancer of the uterus.

Content and metabolism of bone tissue. Bone consists of a large number of minerals, closely combined with each other and with bone protein. Yet conventional mineral treatment of osteoporosis has largely been limited to calcium. The recommendations of the AHA and some Heart Foundations to reduce milk intake because of its supposed high cholesterol content (despite the fact that these recommendations have been proved wrong), has aggravated matters.

Possibly the reason why the concentration on calcium has been uppermost is because 99% of the total body calcium is in bone. But then similarly, of the total minerals in the body, 80-88% of phosphate, 50-60% of magnesium, 80% carbonate, 60-70% manganese, 30-40% sodium, 30% zinc, and more than 50% fluoride is also in bone. All these minerals must and do play an active role in bone formation and metabolism.

Magnesium is particularly important as half the bone magnesium is part of the apatite crystal in bone. Without magnesium bone cannot form this necessary hard core (Aikawa J.K., *Magnesium: Its Biological Significance*, 1981). The National Institutes of Health workshop on osteoporosis in 1987 recommended a daily intake of 1 500 mg of calcium per day by postmenopausal women to prevent osteoporosis, but even a dosage of 3 000 mg failed to have the desired effect. However, in a study in California, 19 postmenopausal women on a diet (high in minerals) plus multimicronutrient tablets containing 500 mg of calcium and 600 mg of magnesium per day, showed a considerable improvement in osteoporosis, even without hormone treatment (*J Reproductive Med* 1990; 35: 503-7).

Once more, osteoporosis, postmenopausal or otherwise, is another example of a modern Western metabolic disease. All methods of processing food will have to be reviewed if this condition is to be prevented in any way. In the meantime an appropriate micronutrient diet and supplementation with high magnesium and calcium content has to be applied. And then there is every reason to believe that we can dispense with female hormones. Why not? Our mothers of old did, without any problems.

Sex Organ and Hormone Disturbances

Probably the oldest application of prostaglandin treatment lies in this field. Intravenous and intra-amniotic PGE2 and PGF1 increase uterus tone with resultant pregnant uterus contractions to initiate a late pregnancy (and cause an early abortion).

It also plays a role in the female menstrual cycle by stimulating the brain's hypothalamus to help the ovary develop the corpus luteum, necessary for pregnancy.

Most of the prostaglandins are present in semen where they have several functions, PGE2 stimulating motility and PGF2 inhibiting it. Numerous studies have indicated that sperm counts amongst persons of Western societies have decreased, e.g. Scotland, where a decrease of 30% has occurred over the last 22 years (*BMJ* 1996; 312: 467-71).

The effect of prostaglandin imbalance on smooth muscle can be the cause of dysmenorrhoea (painful contractions during menstruation), the premenstrual syndrome, pre-eclampsia, complications of pregnancy, diabetes in pregnancy and infertility in women (Curtis-Prior, 1988). Frequently the imbalance causes increased oestrogen and decreased progesterone leading to amenorrhoea, sterility, irregular menstruation, possibly myomata and an increased incidence of uterus cancer.

The clinician is frequently faced with the severe problem of how to rebalance the hormones without aggravating the condition. After numerous unsuccessful hormonal manipulations, treatment frequently ends in a premature hysterectomy. It would have been to the patient's advantage if therapy with micronutrients, diet and supplementation, with a particularly high vitamin B6 content, was attempted. Vitamin B6's oldest therapeutic application has been in premenstrual tension, with excellent results.

Another problem of a high oestrogen level arise in relation to the amino acid **tryptophane**, which has a choice of two metabolic pathways, either to **seretonin**, the natural antidepressant, or to **nicotinic acid**, the vitamin with over 420 enzyme commitments.

Increased oestrogen stimulates the reaction towards the nicotinic acid pathway, decreasing the seretonin and thereby causing a depression (*Am J Clin Nutr* 1975; 28: 146-56). This is frequently seen after childbirth when a woman still has a high oestrogen level and nothing to work on. Increased vitamin B6 treatment will increase the seretonin and thus relieve depression.

Strokes or Brain Blood Vessel Lesions

This was a very common condition a few decades back, but since the improved control of high blood pressure the incidence has declined. Strokes can lead either to sudden death or to a prolonged illness with one-sided paralysis, and sometimes partial improvement. The prevalence is much higher in blacks than in whites. It has a high incidence of death in diabetics (*Am J Med* 1996; 100: 517-23).

The aim must therefore be prevention. It has lately become abundantly clear that the most important cause of cerebral thrombosis is an increase in blood **homocysteine,** 2.3 times more important than high blood pressure (Clarke, *NEJM* 1991; 324: 1149-55). The method of prevention is thus obvious: a high genetic micronutrient diet with multimicronutrient supplementation.

Deep Venous Thrombosis (DVT)

Many people suffer from this condition, especially in the calf of the leg. It is often accompanied by a local infection when it becomes acute thrombophlebitis. It can commonly develop from a forced stay in bed after major surgery, but not in all cases. In 50% of cases there may be no symptoms at all. Frequently it may indicate a cancer somewhere in the body.

Though bed rest and heat may be sufficient in some cases, the conventional treatment is anticoagulants with intravenous heparin, switching to long-term therapy with warfarin. The latter treatment must be well controlled with numerous laboratory coagulative investigations.

However, the same article referred to under "Strokes" has indicated that a high blood **homocysteine** plays an important role in DVT. Consequently an appropriate diet and micronutrient supplementation can act as prevention and treatment. It would be advisable to continue with the warfarin for a while but experience has proved that the thrombus will disappear shortly with micronutrients.

Chronic Fatigue Syndrome or Myalgic Encephalomyelitis (ME)

No new illness has baffled the medical profession more than this condition. Authorities argue whether chronic fatigue syndrome and ME are one and the same disease. Some declare that you cannot talk of ME unless a brain lesion is present.

The history of ME goes back as far as 1948 when, in an Icelandic epidemic, it was called "akureyri disease". The usual history of this disease, to all appearances, is a slow recovery from an acute viral infection, for example such as a virus heart muscle infection (myocarditis), as described by Dr Karen Prince, a sufferer (*BMJ* 1994; 308: 1300). In some cases evidence of an immunological disorder is present (hypersensitivity tests) and in others not.

Usually frequent relapses take place, possibly due to reactivated virus infections, with both mental and physical exhaustion, which is relieved by rest. The symptoms, besides fatigue, are usually depression, anxiety, sleep disorders, fibromyalgia (pains in the body muscles) and hyperventilation (uncontrolled deep breathing). Frequently the sufferers lose much in terms of family, career, social life and financial position.

The present prevalence of the disease is estimated as high as 3% in certain general practices in Britain, while other estimates are 1,3 per 1 000.

Though psychiatric disorders may be present, they are no more so than are found in studies of patients with other medical conditions such as cancer. The severity of the physical symptoms can vary from mild tiredness and headaches to a severe inability to walk.

The eventual outcome of the disease is difficult to predict, but a reasonable estimate is that 40% of patients will follow a fluctuating course, 15-20% will remain severely affected, 5-10% will deteriorate, and only 35% will improve to the point of apparent total recovery (Sandra Howes, *BMJ* 1994; 308: 1300).

Once the diagnosis has been made the best procedure is to join an ME Association. They advocate an appropriate period of rest and convalescence, followed by a carefully paced increase in both physical and mental activity. Of course, certain persons, such as executives and businesspeople, may not have the time to follow fully the Association's advice, but they have an excellent alternative.

Treatment with a high multimicronutrient diet and supplements have excellent results while the patient is on therapy. This may lead to enough improvement to suggest a cure. The test will, however, be whether the improvement or cure is sustained when multimicronutrients are decreased.

This is not strictly speaking a modern metabolic disease due to micronutrient loss in the diet, but one could speculate that the genetic high micronutrient diet of the past could have warded off the virus infection and/or prevented the fatigue symptoms.

Alzheimer's Disease

This is the commonest cause of dementia. Dementia is defined as a form of insanity consisting of mental feebleness rather than derangement. In the United Kingdom it affects 400 000 people, with about 18 000 of these below retirement age. Some already develop it in their thirties (*BMJ* 1993; 307: 779-82).

The development of the disease, first described by Alois Alzheimer in 1906 in a 50-year-old woman, varies considerably. In some it is familial, in most it is sporadic. Some have an early onset, others a late onset. In some the disease progresses rapidly over three to four years, others have slow progression over 20 years. Usually memory is the first function to go, and sometimes problems with language. In others, loss of executive-type functions, such as planning and organisation are early signs.

According to studies the prevalence of Alzheimer's is low in blacks, both American and Nigerian. It has been stated to be associated only with technically advanced societies (*Am J Psychiatry*; 1996 152: 1485-92).

As yet, no conventional treatment can permanently halt, reverse or prevent the disease. The main aim is to preserve the quality of life as long as possible. Usually the diagnosis is made as long as two to three years after the initial symptoms, and death is usually within ten years.

Relatives want to know what the risk is of inheriting the disease. In first-degree relatives the risk will be approximately fourfold greater in comparison with the general public if the disease develops before 65 years, and double if the patient developed it after 65 years. When there is a strong history of dominant familial Alzheimer's the risk is 50%.

As in hypercholesterolaemia, Alzheimer's also has a dominant genetic form and a recessive or less serious form. The dominant form always affects younger persons in their thirties or forties. Typically, up to half of the patients have a family history, but only 5-10% have a true dominant disease. About 80% of the latter is due to a gene fault in chromosome 14, and the rest in chromosome I, but the cause of the late onset type is less clear with a variation in apo-lipoprotein E which binds a protein known as amyloid (*Science* 1995; 269: 917-8). The latter could be in chromosome 21.

The key faults in Alzheimer's are abnormal nerve-fibril "tangles" and senile plaques in different parts of the brain causing an abnormal form of a protein known as **tau**. Normally this tau maintains certain microtubes in the brain for normal function. The senile plaque consists of nerve particles clustered around the above-mentioned amyloid. Some unknown factor converts normal amyloid into an abnormal insoluble amyloid which increases in the brain tissue, causing many of the nerve symptoms of Alzheimer's. Tau protein can now be measured in the spinal fluid at average values of 279 ng/l as compared to mean values of 88 ng/l in brain stroke lesions (*J Neurology, Neurosurgery and Psychiatry* 1995; 59: 280-3).

Most of the neurotransmitters are decreased in Alzheimer's, but the most affected is **acetylcholine**, the major transmitter for memory. To date, the only drug approved for the treatment of the disease is Tactrine, whose main action is to block acetylcholinesterase, the enzyme which destroys acetylcholine. The action of acetylcholinesterase can, however, be diverted into another direction by at least three micronutrients: magnesium, nicotinic acid and sodium. Tactrine provides some benefit for certain patients but has gastro-intestinal and liver side effects. Aluminium, once considered an important factor in Alzheimer's, has been disproved as a cause.

Once again micronutrients could come to the rescue, not to cure but to relieve. High dosages of multimicronutrients have been shown to relieve symptoms considerably and this treatment must be applied diligently.

Here, too, Alzheimer Associations and Societies are in existence to aid and advise not only the patients, but also their close relatives.

Carbohydrate Craving Depression

Most people pick up mass during the winter months and lose it again as summer appears, a state believed to be due to the colder season stimulating the appetite "to fatten the body against the cold". But this is not the whole story. A large percentage, perhaps the majority, of people are especially stimulated to eat carbohydrate foods and snacks with a high sugar content. They are frequently accused of having a "sweet tooth". This condition has been named carbohydrate craving syndrome (Wurtman R.J. et al., *Scientific American*, Jan. 1989).

A biochemical substance, **melatonin**, has been found to play a dominant role in this condition. Melatonin, a substance sensitive to light, especially sunlight, and a stimulant for skin pigmentation, varies in blood and tissue concentrations during day and night, and increases as the afternoon sun fades. At this time of day it causes a craving for sweet carbohydrate-rich foods, accompanied by a mood depression. Significantly, it is formed from seretonin, already discussed under depression (Fig 10.1).

↓ decreased concentration; ↑ increased concentration.

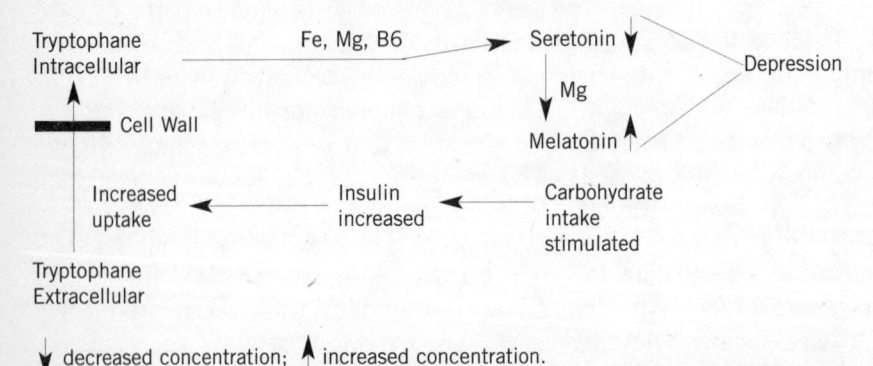

Fig 10.1. Carbohydrate craving depression. Increased melatonin increases depression. To counteract this, seretonin in the brain must be increased. This occurs via the mechanism of carbohydrate stimulation to increase insulin, which facilitates increased uptake of intracellular tryptophane.

Being sensitive to sunlight it increases earlier in the shorter winter days, thereby stimulating the carbohydrate craving earlier in the afternoon. This all has a reason: the high sugar-containing carbohydrate intake stimulates the pancreas to secrete more insulin. The latter is known to stimulate the uptake of tryptophane into the cells (also in the brain), thereby increasing the previously low seretonin. This alleviates the symptoms of depression but, unhappily, increases the mass. Perhaps this is the reason why fat people always appear cheerful and are seldom depressed.

So a vicious circle develops, with increased mass in winter, intensifying every new winter season. Again the primary cause is almost certainly the dietary shortage of iron, magnesium and vitamin B6, a condition which can be reversed by the genetic micronutrient diet and micronutrient supplementation.

Mitral Valve Prolapse (MVP) and Depression

Mitral valve prolapse became known many years ago when a Johannesburg cardiologist, Dr Barlow, discovered a unique heart murmur in young to middle-aged persons. The murmur is due to a billowing-like weakening of the heart's mitral valve wall, likened to a yacht's sail in the wind. Usually the patient suffers little discomfort, and most often the diagnosis is made by chance during a routine examination. The symptoms vary from slight shortness of breath and irregular heartbeats to acute collapse and tachycardia (very fast heartbeat and pulse). Very occasionally surgery is necessary to heal the valve.

Through research by Dr Will Davis, a physician in Johannesburg, his son Dr Henry Davis, a medically qualified geneticist, Prof George Gericke, a paediatrician-geneticist, and Dr Sieg Bissbort, a biochemical geneticist (the last three all from Pretoria) the chemical cause of the condition has been discovered (see Fig 10.2). The primary fault lies with polymorphism of the enzyme **methionine adenosyl transmethylase (MAT)**, leading to decreased metabolism of the pathway to homocysteine and cysteine. Cysteine is an important amino acid in muscle and tissue protein. Its decreased formation leads to mitral valve prolapse and hyperextension of arm and leg joints (X-legs). At the same time fewer methyl groups are available to stimulate noradrenaline to form adrenaline, and depression develops.

The effect on the patient is MVP, joint hyperextension, double-jointedness, X-legs and mental depression. It has been estimated that approximately as high as 17% of persons in Western societies have MVP.

172 • A BLUEPRINT FOR BETTER HEALTH

```
➤ Methionine ─────────────────────────── essential amino acid
  Mg │ Methionine
     │ Adenosyl ──────────────────────── fault lies with
     │ Transmethylase                     polymorphic
  K  ▼                                    form
  S Adenosyl methionine
      ┌──── Noradrenaline                 causes depression
      │        Ca ─┐
      │            ▼
   Methyl       Vanyl man- ──────────┐    decreases
                 delic acid          │    symptoms
   donor           ▲
      │         Ca ─┘
      └──➤ Adrenaline ──────────────────── causes excitation
      ▼
  S Adenosyl homocysteine
      ▼
  ─ Homocysteine ─────────────────────── decreased, free
      │                                   of atherosclerosis
      │ B6
      ▼
  Cystathhionine
      │
      │ B6
      ▼
  Cysteine ──────────────────────────── decreased, an important
                                         tissue amino acid
```

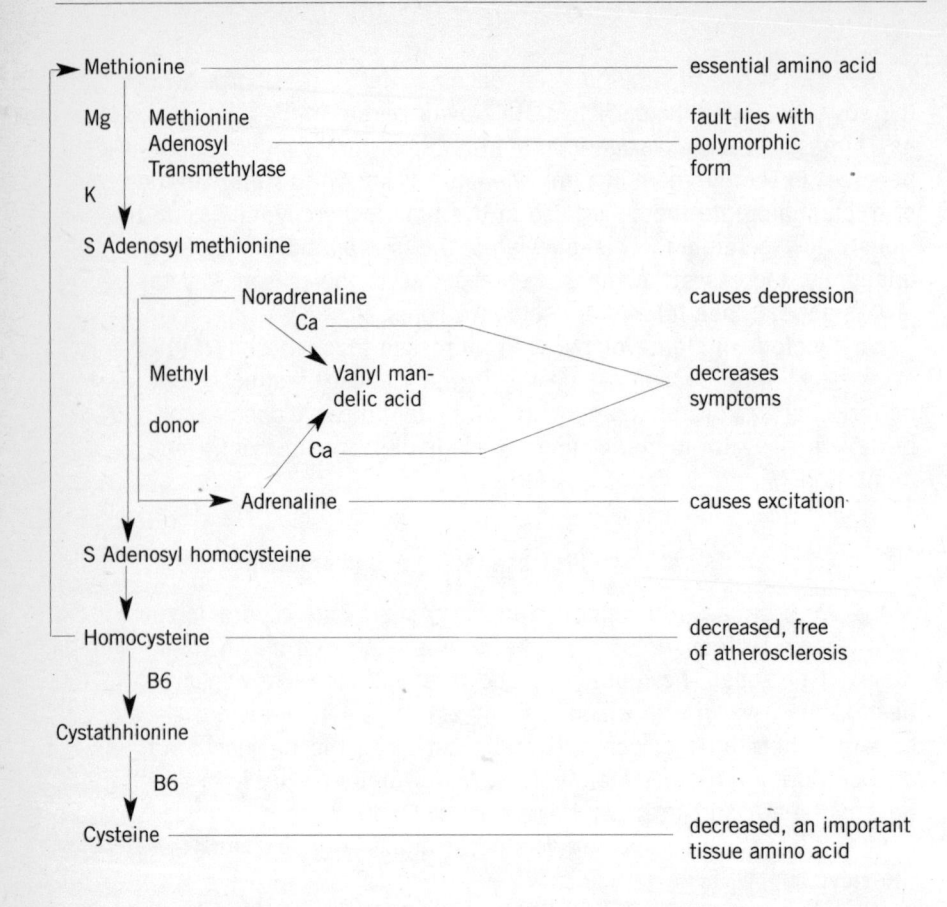

Fig 10.2. Mitral valve prolapse (Barlow's syndrome). Diagrammatic presentation of methionine adenosyl transferase polymorphism with resultant clinical signs. Note that the main therapy is administering of magnesium, calcium and potassium.

Fortunately, due to reduced homocysteine formation, the danger of heart attacks is considerably decreased. These persons are frequently very tall, thin, long-fingered and long-toed, similar to those suffering from a congenital condition known as Marfan's syndrome. It has been suggested that Abraham Lincoln was a Marfan. More likely, he was a mitral valve prolapse.

Note once more the important role of micronutrients. Undoubtedly a dietary loss thereof must aggravate the symptoms. The author has the experience of a single case in which the genetic micronutrient diet plus supplements changed the rumbling roar of an MVP murmur to a faint pulsating whisper.

Tourette Syndrome

This fascinating syndrome, which sometimes has tragic results, was first described by Tourette, and is now firmly established (Comings D.E., *Am J Human Genetics*, 1989). Numerous and varying psychological symptoms are noted from childhood to adulthood, leading to serious behavioural and social problems. Characteristic is a restless tic (habitual spasms noted in the body – remember the murderer in Alfred Hitchcock's *Psycho*?), accompanied by other behavioural abnormalities.

The problem starts during school-going years: high energy (hyperactivity), easily distracted, loss of concentration, constant unnecessary nagging, always seeking something new (impulsivity) and getting one's own way (compulsivity). These children are frequently told they are lazy and underachievers. Consequently they feel helpless and frustrated, setting the stage for future catastrophes, such as lawlessness, sexual promiscuity, alcohol abuse and drug dependency – especially if there is lack of discipline. Depression is common amongst them.

Carried through to adulthood, many show high-energy creativity with an acute awareness of other people's feelings (a good business sense sometimes used to the detriment of gullible persons), an unusual sensitivity to colour, form and shape (artists, writers, poets), exceptional musical talent, tenacity which allows them to get their own way (lawyers, business people). Many of them are looked upon by the community as cranks.

Tourette's syndrome is probably fairly common (1/100 in USA boys), which means that 13% of the general population are carriers. Many do not need treatment at all, while the rest can be successfully treated with a dopamine receptor antagonist (Shapiro A.K. et al., *Pediatrics*, 1987). It is obvious that micronutrients must be supplemented, especially magnesium, calcium and potassium, to facilitate control of the varied symptoms.

The fault lies with a polymorphic genetic overstimulation of an enzyme, tryptophane dioxygenase, which increases the formation of quinolate, a substance stimulating excitability. At present only a few laboratories in the world are able to estimate this enzyme for diagnostic purposes. No doubt, as the importance of this enzyme becomes generally known, the laboratory diagnosis of Tourette's syndrome will become simplified.

This is another example of a medical condition in which genetic and environmental factors combine to produce a complex neuropsychiatric disorder (*JAMA* 1995; 273: 498-501).

Acne

If old portraits and paintings are an indication, acne was either absent or extremely rare before 1880, even granted that artists would smooth over the blemishes of their clients' skins. Even the cruellest cartoonists of those days, such as Toulouse-Lautrec, though emphasising warts and moles, never depicted anything that looked like acne. Also, among rural blacks the condition is absent.

Modern conventional treatment of acne, which includes rice bran oil, antibiotics, oestrogen and cortisol, suggests an important role for unrefined foods containing maximum micronutrients in the battle against decreased immunity. The present most accepted form of treatment is retinoids, which are formed from vitamin A. Like vitamin E, vitamin A is removed from practically all refined foods. Because these vitamins are fat soluble, they are removed to lengthen the shelf life of certain foodstuffs. However, the treatment effect of these retinoids is so potent that women who become pregnant while using them, have a risk of producing abnormal babies.

For a very long time patients have been warned to avoid greasy foods, as for example in the book *Diseases and Remedies* published in 1901. Yet the AHA advises that polyunsaturates are beneficial to heart disease, so oily food intake has increased in the last two to three decades. Could this be the cause of the obvious increase of acne in teenagers?

Low levels of zinc have been found in those suffering from advanced acne (Michaelson G. et al., *Arch Dermatology*, 1977). Although other vitamins and minerals were not investigated at the same time, it can be presumed that if zinc is low, other micronutrients will also be low.

Acne calls for a genetic micronutrient diet from very early on in life. Supplementation with zinc, magnesium, vitamin C, vitamin E and vitamin A is advised.

Parkinson's Disease

First described by James Parkinson in 1917, this is a neurological disease affecting the nervous system in middle-aged or elderly people. It affects 1.5% of Western populations over 65 years of age. There is a definite gradual increase in cases diagnosed, although this may be partly due to the population living longer.

Four typical symptoms are noted: bradykinesis (slow movements), rigidity, tremor (typically a "pill-rolling" effect of the fingers, especially at rest), and a characteristic walk and body position (stumbling, leaning forward). Although the intelligence initially remains normal, conversation is difficult, causing frustration to both patient and listener. Later a measure of depression and psychological disorder occurs.

It is now clear that the cause of the condition is a decrease in **dopamine,** a neurotransmitter that carries impulses in the brain. This is probably due to environmental and body-formed nerve poisons, and not to a virus, as once was believed. These poisons are toxic substances as well as oxidised products formed in the brain (Elizan T.S. et al., *Arch Neurol*, 1989). These oxidised products develop when a shortage of vitamins A and D occur.

Conventional treatment has been to administer a forerunner of dopamine known as levodopa. It is useless administering dopamine as it cannot cross into the brain, whereas levodopa can cross the brain barrier. The important fact is that the compound causing the conversion of levodopa to dopamine in the brain is vitamin B6. The loss of the highly important vitamins B6, A and E in the refined Western diets must therefore play a significant role in the aggravation of Parkinson's disease.

Dental Caries

Dental caries (tooth decay) and pyorrhoea (gum infection) are the most prevalent chronic dental diseases in the developed world. Until lately, certain primitive peoples such as older Eskimos, some Pacific Islanders, Greenlanders and rural Africans, who lived in isolated areas under natural conditions, suffered far less from dental caries than people in the more developed areas (Schaeffer O., *Nutrition Today*, 1971).

Usually an infection due to a bacteria, streptococcus mutans, is present, leading to the production of acids. The latter causes decalcification of the tooth enamel. A pH of below 5.5 is critical for the development of caries. The active bacteria apparently prefer sucrose (refined crystal sugar), but they also act in the presence of other sugars, including honey. It is the sticky or gluey confectioneries that are far more capable of causing caries than a solution of sugar, such as in tea, coffee or cool drinks (*Krause and Mahon Textbook*, 1984).

The highest concentrations of sugars in popular foods are in commercial cool drinks (Coke 9.2 teaspoons per 12 ounces; Sprite 9.0 teaspoons per 12 ounces), cranberry sauce (11.7 teaspoons per half a cup), and fruit yoghurt (7.5 teaspoons per eight ounces) (*Krause and Mahon Textbook*, 1984).

Frequent eating also plays a detrimental role. Consequently confectionary snacks are to be discouraged.

A deficiency of vitamins A, B-complex, C and D in the diet have all, at some time or another, been blamed for some form of caries. Similarly minerals, particularly calcium and phosphorous, are most important in preventing caries. But the role of magnesium, manganese and other trace minerals in the formation of teeth and prevention of caries must not be underestimated. Fluoride in drinking water and toothpaste has proved its preventative role in dental caries.

CHAPTER 11

IN CONCLUSION . . .

The little present must not be allowed to wholly elbow the great past out of view.
ANDREW LANG (1844-1912)

In judging any statements or claims made by medical science, it is as well to look for prejudice and arrogance (in ourselves as well as in the writer), and to be alert for commercially influenced opinions. And if the reader has, at times, been understandably confused by the bewildering number of facts and arguments in the previous pages, I urge him or her not to be deterred from taking steps to better health. After all, few battles have been fought more bitterly than those conducted through the pages of medical journals, but I hope that I have given a clear indication where the hope for future health lies.

During the last century, one Ignaz Semmelweis committed suicide when he was universally mocked for his suggestion that doctors should wash their hands before examining expectant mothers. The moral of the story is that we should not be too hasty in rejecting new ideas in the field of medical science.

As I hope I have satisfactorily demonstrated in these pages, the history of heart disease is paralleled by that of all other contemporary metabolic diseases, and research points to the same basic cause: a loss of micronutrients due to food-processing procedures. A number of metabolic diseases arise from genetic factors, but sufferers from these, too, can derive great benefit from micronutrient diets and therapy.

As I have stressed throughout, among the awesome number of sometimes fatal conditions that threaten us are coronary heart disease, high blood pressure, diabetes mellitus type II, rheumatoid arthritis, cancer, osteoporosis, obesity, spastic colon, depression, acne, auto-immune diseases, allergies and dental caries.

Based on both documented research and personal experience, I can only advise, indeed plead, with the public to follow a genetic micronutrient diet, with micronutrient supplementation where necessary, for both the prevention and treatment of all Western metabolic diseases.

APPENDIX A:

TABLES OF FOODSTUFFS CONTAINING MAGNESIUM, VITAMIN B6, ZINC AND FIBRE

Values reported in descending concentrations for magnesium.

Legumes	mg Mg /100 g	mg B6 /100 g	mg Zn /100 g	g fibre /100 g
Beans, white, kidney, dry, raw	164	0.580	2.80	21.6
Chick peas, dried, raw	160	?	?	15.0
Peas, dried, raw	130	0.130	4.00	11.9
Lentils, raw	73	0.606	3.13	11.8
Baked beans	31	0.120	0.70	7.3
Soya beans	?	0.180	3.52	4.9

Cereals	mg Mg /100 g	mg B6 /100 g	mg Zn /100 g	g fibre /100 g
Bran, wheat, unprocessed	520	1.380	16.20	44.0
All-Bran Flakes	373	0.830	8.40	29.9
Wheat germ, toasted, plain	240	0.730	12.50	20.3
Oats, uncooked	148	0.120	3.07	5.6
Raisin Bran	129	?	?	10.6
ProNutro	125	1.300	3.00	15.1
Weet-Bix	120	0.240	2.10	12.7
Maize meal, white, whole kernel, raw	107	0.400	2.00	9.1
Maltabella, dry (sorghum)	102	?	2.30	2.0
Rye, crispbread (Ryvita)	100	0.290	3.10	11.7
Muesli	100	0.140	2.20	7.4
Bread, whole-wheat	88	0.147	2.32	8.9
Maize meal, white, unsifted, raw	88	?	1.74	8.1
Bread, brown	58	0.080	1.38	5.3
Special K	55	0.160	1.90	0.8
Rice, cooked, brown	54	0.231	?	1.3
Bread, white	37	0.041	1.05	2.8
Cookies, commercial, plain	33	0.061	0.61	5.6
Maize meal, white, super, raw	28	?	0.61	3.2
Oats, cooked	24	0.020	0.49	0.9
Spaghetti bolognaise	19	0.108	1.66	0.6
Macaroni and cheese	16	0.041	0.80	0
Corn, puffed	15	?	0.46	0.6

Cornflakes, plain	12	0,065	0,28	2,8
Cake, butter, plain, home-made	10	0,072	0,52	1,0
Rice, cooked, white	4	0,046	0,36	0,7

Nuts	mg Mg /100 g	mg B6 /100 g	mg Zn /100 g	g fibre /100 g
Sunflower seeds, kernels, dried	354	1.250	5.06	4.2
Almonds, dried, blanched	286	0.101	3.16	6.1
Hazelnuts, dried, blanched	285	0.612	2.40	9.8
Pumpkin seeds, whole, roasted	262	?	10.30	35.9
Cashew nuts, dried, roasted	260	0.256	5.60	0.7
Brazil nuts, dried, shelled	225	0.251	4.59	9.5
Peanuts, roasted	188	0.389	6.62	8.3
Walnuts, dried, shelled	169	0.558	2.73	6.5
Pistachio nuts, dried	158	?	1.34	1.9
Pecan nuts	128	0.188	5.47	1.6
Coconut meat, raw	32	0.054	1.10	12.4
Chestnuts, fresh, peeled	30	0.330	0.49	6.8

Meat	mg Mg /100 g	mg B6 /100 g	mg Zn /100 g	g fibre /100 g
Pork grilled, loin chop	29	0.460	2.92	0
Mutton, roasted, leg	28	0.220	5.30	0
Veal, roasted	28	0.320	?	0
Beef, grilled, sirloin	22	0.330	5.50	0
Chicken, boiled	20	0.270	1.35	0
Liver, beef, fried	19	0.520	4.30	0
Tongue, ox, cooked	16	0.090	?	0
Ham, cooked/canned	13	0.320	1.83	0
Frankfurter, beef and pork	10	0.130	1.84	0

Fruit	mg Mg /100 g	mg B6 /100 g	mg Zn /100 g	g fibre /100 g
Avocado	39	0.280	0.42	2.1
Dates, dried, raw	35	0.192	0.29	7.9
Fruit rolls, dried	33	0.144	0.42	9.7
Raisins, raw	33	0.249	0.27	7.3
Bananas, raw	29	0.578	0.16	3.0
Granadilla	29	?	?	15.9

Olives, green, pickled	22	0.020	?	4.4
Kiwi fruit, raw	19	?	0.17	2.8
Fig, raw	17	0.113	0.15	3.4
Prunes, dried, raw	14	0.260	0.08	14.2
Pineapples, raw	14	0.087	0.08	1.5
Fruit salad, fresh	12	0.102	0.10	1.9
Mandarine (nartjie)	12	0.067	0.10	1.9
Watermelon, raw	11	0.144	0.07	0.3
Guava, raw	10	0.143	0.23	5.6
Orange, raw	10	0.060	0.07	2.0
Pawpaw, raw	10	0.019	0.07	0.9
Mango, raw	9	0.134	0.04	1.6
Apricot, raw	8	0.054	0.26	2.1
Grapefruit, raw	8	0.042	0.07	0.6
Plum, raw	7	0.081	0.10	2.0
Peach, raw	7	0.018	0.14	1.2
Pear, raw	6	0.018	0.12	2.5
Grapes, raw	6	0.110	0.05	1.7
Apple, raw	5	0.048	0.04	3.1
Vegetables	mg Mg /100 g	mg B6 /100 g	mg Zn /100 g	g fibre /100 g
Spinach, cooked	87	0.242	0.76	2.7
Potato chips, commercial crisps	60	0.513	1.07	1.3
Peas, fresh/frozen, cooked/canned	39	0.216	1.19	5.7
Beetroot, cooked	37	0.031	0.25	1.3
Potato, baked-in-jacket	27	0.347	0.32	2.5
Beans, green, cooked	25	0.056	0.36	3.9
Pumpkin and squash, cooked	24	0.065	0.39	1.6
Potato, boiled with skin	20	0.269	0.27	1.2
Carrot, raw	15	0.240	0.20	2.5
Cabbage, raw	15	0.095	0.18	2.2
Cauliflower, raw	14	0.230	0.18	2.1
Pepper, green, raw	14	0.164	0.18	0.9
Brinjal, cooked	13	0.086	0.15	3.1
Tomato, raw	11	0.048	0.11	1.5
Cucumber, raw	11	0.052	0.23	0.5
Mushroom, raw	10	0.097	0.73	2.5
Onions, raw	10	0.157	0.18	1.7
Lettuce, raw	9	0.040	0.22	1.5

Miscellaneous	mg Mg /100 g	mg B6 /100 g	mg Zn /100 g	g fibre /100 g
Cocoa, dry, powder	520	0.07	6.90	?
Chocolate, bitter	292	?	2.30?	
Marzipan	259	?	2.58	6.0
Curry powder	254	?	4.05	16.3
Yeast, baker's, dried	230	2.000	8,0	21.9
Dried fruit sweets	23	0.081	0.30	6.9
Coconut ice	18	0.060	0.40	4.7
Macaroni, cooked, and whole-wheat	18	0.010	0.30	?
Sugar, brown	15	0	?	0
Beer, average	9	0.027	0.01	0
Honey, strained	2	?	?	0
Margarine, polyunsaturated	1	0	0	0
Sugar, white	0	0	?	0

From: "Composition of foods", *Agricultural Handbook No 8*, 1975 and 1984, USA; Gous E. and Langenhoven M.L. *Food composition tables* (2nd edition), Parow, South African Medical Research Council, 1986.

APPENDIX B

FOOD PRODUCTION EFFECTS ON VITAMING B6 CONTENT OF FOODS

Food	mg B6 /100 g	% Decrease
Rice, brown, raw	0.55	
Rice, white, precooked	0.034	-94%
Kale, raw	0.30	
Kale, frozen	0.19	-37%
Spinach, raw	0.28	
Spinach, frozen	0.19	-32%
Potatoes, raw	0.25	
Potatoes, canned	0.10	-60%
Brussels sprouts, raw	0.23	
Brussels sprouts, frozen	0.15	-35%

Food	mg B6 /100 g	% Decrease
Sweet potatoes, raw	0.660	
Sweet potatoes, canned	0.218	-70%
Cauliflower, fresh	0.21	
Cauliflower, frozen	0.19	-10%
Broccoli, raw	0.195	
Broccoli, frozen	0.15	-23%
Peas, raw	0.18	
Peas, canned	0.05	-72%
Beans, lima, raw	0.17	
Beans, lima, canned	0.09	-47%
Asparagus, raw	0.16	
Asparagus, canned	0.06	-62%
Carrots, raw	0.15	
Carrots, canned	0.03	-80%
Mushrooms, raw	0.125	
Mushrooms, canned	0.056	-55%
Beans, snap, raw	0.08	
Beans, snap, frozen	0.07	-13%
Beans, snap, canned	0.04	-50%
Raspberries, raw	0.06	
Raspberries, frozen	0.038	-37%
Strawberries, raw	0.055	
Strawberries, frozen	0.043	-22%
Plums, raw	0.052	
Plums, canned	0.027	-48%
Orange juice, fresh	0.04	
Orange juice, canned	0.035	-13%
Orange juice, frozen	0.028	-20%
Peaches, raw	0.024	
Peaches, canned	0.019	-21%
Peaches, frozen	0.018	-25%

Reference: Gruberg E.R. and Raymond S., *Beyond Cholesterol. Vitamin B6, Arteriosclerosis, and Your Heart,* New York: St Martin's Press, 1981.

INDEX

A
acetaldehyde dehydrogenase, polymorphism 27
acetylcholine 153
  in Alzheimers 169
acne 134f, 174
additives, effect on food 89
adenosyl homocysteine 63f
  methionine 63f
adipostat 157
African, diets, breakfast 121
  other meals 123
Ahrens, Prof Edward 67
Aids 146, 148
alcohol, blood, safe limits 107-108
  dehydrogenase, polymorphism 27f, 28
  maximum for efficient liver metabolism 107
alcoholism, incidence 107
aldosterone, negative effects of statins 81
alpha-linolenic acid 134f, 145f
Alzheimer's disease 47, 168
amenorrhoea 166
American Council of Science and Health 72
American Heart Association (AHA), diet recommendations 50
  criticisms 50-51
American physician study, homocysteine 78
Amerindians, genetic race 22
animal fats, consumption, USA 99f
  genetic 125
Anitschkow 49, 59, 71
antihypertensive drugs, side effects 137
antioxidants 91, 92, 92f, 94f
appetite suppressors 159
arachidonic acid 41, 41f, 134f
arteriography, coronary 73
Ascherio, Dr Albert 53
Asian, genetic race 23
aspirin 74
asthma 146
atherosclerosis, final common pathway 100, 101
  heart disease, "new" disease 31
Australian Aborigines, genetic race 22
auto-immune diseases 134f, 145f
avocados, diet 120
Axelrod, Dr Abe 147

B
bananas, diet 120
Barker's syndrome, childhood risk factors 84
Barlow's syndrome 171
barbecues 126
Beauty Queen diet 159
beef, fat content 20t
betaine 63f
beverages, diet 119
Bible 20
blood pressure, normal 135
  high 135
body mass index (BMI) 156
Bogdarich, Walt, inaccurate cholesterol estimations 70
Boyd, Dr W.C., genetic races 22
bran, digestive 117, 157
  content 118t
Braunwald, Prof Eugene 100
bread, flour, content 118t
  stabilisers 118
  transfatty acids 118, 119
  types 118
breakfast, examples 120-121
breast cancer gene 151
Brett, Dr Allan 71
British Diabetic Association 141
Bronte-Stewart, Dr 53
Brusis, Dr 62, 97, 97t
Burkitt Dr 156
  and Trowell 32, 46t
business lunches 122
butter 52, 90, 119
  fat content 20t
  vs margarine consumption 1986 54, 55t

C
Caerphilly study 52, 56, 119

calcium, in bone 165
Cambridge study, milk 119
cancer 148
  breast 151
  colon, red meat 125
  dietary factors 150
  lung 151
    smoking 105
    diet 106
  prostate 152
  prostaglandin function 44f
  PUFAs, danger 149
  therapy, secondary effects 148
  world trends 149
canning, food, effects 89
Cape Peninsula Study on cholesterol 83
carbohydrate craving depression 170
carbohydrates 26, 25f
  complex 51
  substituted for saturated fatty acids 55
cardiovascular, prostaglandins 44f
cat family 42
causes of death, International List 31
  coronary heart disease 31
cellular functions, prostaglandins 44f
cerebral thrombosis, homocysteine 78
cheese, diet 122
chicken, diet 126
chips, dried, potato, diet 127
cholesterol, blood estimations, inaccuracy 70
  blood, opinions of physicians 68
  blood values 48
  concentrations in food 125t
  decreased, personal experience 98
  dietary, little increase in blood 54, 95
  dietary, on atherosclerosis 101-102, 101f
  difficult lowering of values 83
  esters 51, 51f, 61, 61t, 95, 101f, 102
  high density (HDL) 60, 61f, 61, 95
  low density (LDL) 60, 61f, 61, 95
  molecule, negative effects of statins 81
  normal values 68, 69f
  not increased by saturated fats 97
  setting sun, moon and darkness 55, 56f
  theory and diet, criticisms 71
  total increased, main cause 95, 96
Cholesterol Consensus Development 67
Cholesterol Education Programme 68
Chlamydia pneumoniae, atherosclerosis 84
chromosomes 25f
chromosomal disorders 26
chronic fatigue syndrome 167-168
Cleave, T.L. 45
coffee, diet 119
commerce, role of 56
confectionery, diet 127
conjunctivitis 145
Connor, William, eggs 120
consumer pressure 114
Corday, Dr Eliot 71
coronary artery bypass surgery (CABS) 73
Coronary Primary Prevention Trial (CPPT) 66
coronary heart disease (CHD), treatment 102
corticosteroid therapy, disadvantages
cortisol, negative effects of statins 81
Crohn's disease 145f, 146
cystathionine synthase 63, 63f
cysteine 171

D

data torturing 67
DeBakey, Prof Michael 72
deep venous thrombosis 93, 167
De Lange, cholesterol increased in Javanese 59
delta-6-desaturase 41f, 42, 43, 45, 91
dementia, in Alzheimer's 168
dental caries 134f, 175
deoxyribonucleic acid (DNA) 25, 25f
depression 134f, 153
De Vigneaue, Dr, discovered homocysteine 62
diabetes mellitus 47, 138
  and triglycerides 62
  increase in incidence 31, 138
  insulin-dependent 139
  "new" disease 131, 139
  noninsulin dependent 139
  in South Asian races 140
dibrosoquinone hydroxylase, in hypertension 136
diet, genetic micronutrient 114
diets, ancient 89

diverticulitis 134f
domestication of man 20
  regions of 20
dopamine 153, 153f, 175
Down's syndrome 26
duodenal ulcers, smoking 106
dysmenorrhoea 166

E
East-Central European, genetic race 23
eczema 145
Efamol 40, 41f
eggs 90, 120
eics 42, 43
emergency cardiac units, introduction 31
emphysema 106
endorphins 110
Enig, Dr Mary 98
enzymes, functions 35
  International Congress 35
  total numbers 35
epinephrine 154f
Eskimos 42
essential fatty acids 40, 41f
  prostaglandin pathway 91, 113
Evening Primrose Oil 41f
executive lunch, diet 122
exercise 110, 160

F
familial hypercholesterolaemia, gene therapy 85
fats, content of foods 39t
fatty acids, classification 40t
  content of foods 39t
Fertile Crescent 20
fibre 59, 157
fibroblast growth factors 47
fish, beneficial to man 42
  fatty content 39t
foam cell, formation 100
folic acid 63f
  fortification in USA foods 104
  lessens cleft lips and palate 104
  lessens spina bifida 104
Framingham study 53, 65, 73, 136
  margarine 53
French paradox 108
fruit, diet 119, 122

G
gamma-linolenic acid (GLA) 40, 41f
garlic, diet 128
gastro-intestinal function, prostaglandins 44f
Gemfibrosil (Lopid) 66
genes, heterozygous, polymorphism 90
  major and minor, effects 163
genetic diet 19, 90
  engineering 28
  metabolism 19
  mutations 26
  not complete 90
  races 22-23, 90
glucose metabolism, prostaglandins 44f
gluten allergy 145
gold therapy, for RA 141
grass, fatty acid content 42
Grave's disease, thyroid 146
Greeks, ancient diets 121

H
hamburgers, diet 127
hayfever 145
health, general deterioration 30
Heart Associations 60
heart attacks, total, increases 73
  not lowered by antihypertensive drugs 104
Heart Diet Study 54
Heart Foundations, incorrect advice 51, 165
Helsinki Study 66
heparin, in DVT 167
Hermanus Study 98
Herrman, Paul 114
high blood pressure 134
  conventional treatment 137
  genetics 136
  homocysteine 78
  lowering does not lessen heart attacks 135
hip replacement, athletes 110
Hippocrates 157
  diabetes 138, 139
histamine 148
  methyltransferase 148
Hodgkins, cancer treatment, later cancers 149
homocysteine 63, 63f, 64, 77, 79
  atherosclerosis 93, 101, 101f, 134f

blood clotting 93
blood estimations, problems 79
comparative risk factor 78
discovery 62
effect on membrane binding sites 94f
International Congress 79, 95
homocystinuria 63
Homo Erectus 19
hormones, prostaglandins 44f
human lymphocytic antigens (HLA) 47
 in rheumatoid arthritis 139, 143
Huntingdon's disease 47
hydrogenation of fats 23
3-hydroxy-3-methyl-glutaryl-coenzyme A reductase 80
hypercholesterolaemia, familial (FH) 26
hypertension 134

I
Ignatowski, A.I. 48
immunity 144
 diseases of, classification 144
immunoglobulins 147
Indians, emigrating 127
Indo-Dravidian, diet 127, 123
 genetic race 22
Indonesians, genetic race 22
infertility 166
inflammations, prostaglandins 44f
insulin resistance syndrome 140
International List of Causes of Death 31, 59
Intersalt study, alcohol 108

J
Japanese, immigrants 127
Javanese diets 59
jogging 110

K
Keys, Ancel 49, 53, 59
kidney function, prostaglandins 44f
Kleinefelter syndrome 26
Korean War study 64

L
lactase, abnormalities 26
 polymorphism 27
Laplanders, genetic race 22
leukaemia, lymphatic 152
leukotrienes 41, 41f, 134f

libido, loss due to statins 81
lifespan of man, decreasing 30
lifestyle, heart trials 111
 trials 105
Lincoln, Abraham 172
linoleic acid 96, 101f, 102, 134f, 145f
 formulas 40, 41f, 43
 increases 23
linolenic acid (alpha) 40, 41f
Lipid Research Clinics Coronary (LRP-CPPT) 54
lipid theory 48
lipoproteins, small (a) 47
liver, alcohol 109
Lopid (Gemfibrosil) 66
loss of micronutrients 36

M
macrophages, in atherosclerosis 93, 94f
magnesium 41f, 42, 63f, 64
 antihypertensive action 137
 calming effect 155
 in bone 165
 therapy in heart disease 103
maize, refined 37, 38t
 super, content 116t, 117
 unrefined 37, 38t
maltabella (sorghum) 38t
Mann, Prof Jim, on diabetic diet 141
Marco Polo, pastas 123
margarine, fat content 39t
 formation of 23
 hoax 52
 increases cholesterol and heart attacks 52-53
 Nurses, Health Study 53
mass, losing for health purposes 158
Marfan syndrome 172
mayonnaise, diet 122
McCully, Dr Kilmer 63, 77
meat, red, beef, diet 124, 125t
Mediterranean, diets 24, 76, 76t, 121, 123
 genetic race 22
Melanesian, genetic race 22
melatonin 154f, 170
mendelian disorders 26
metabolic diseases 35f, 45
 advent of 34
 pathways 34, 35f

methionine 63f, 101f, 125t
  discovery, Dr Muller 62
  in meats 125t
methionine adenosyl transmethylase (MAT) 171
methionine-homocysteine pathway 90, 113
micronutrients, additional advantages 104
  cholesterol control 51
  in diet, comparison 129
  in meats 125t
  immune function, congress 147
  loss of 36, 37t
  most important function 34
  loss over years 99f
  stimulating respective enzymes 91
midday meal 121
milk, Caerphilly study 119
  diet 119
  full cream 53, 90, 119
mitral valve prolapse 171
Muller, Dr J.H., discovery of methionine 62
multiple, metabolic disease in persons 104
  sclerosis 47
Multiple Risk Factor Intervention Trial (MRFIT) 54, 65
mutations, enzyme 27
  genetic 24
  1 000 years 24
myalgic encephalomyelitis (ME) 167
myelofibrosis 47, 146
myomata 166

N

nervous system, prostaglandins 44f
neurotransmitters, depression 153
Newburgh and Marsh, Drs 62
niacin (nicotinic acid) 41f, 42
nicotinic acid (niacin) 41f, 42
Nobel prize, for helix structure 24
  for prostaglandins 42
  for steroids 142
noradrenaline 153, 154f
norepinephrine 153
North-West European, genetic race 22, 113

O

oats, bran, content 116t

breakfast food 117
obesity 156
  gene 156
ob-gene 157
oestrogen, negative effect of statins 81
Olestra 85
olive oil, in Mediterranean diets 24, 76, 76t
Oliver, Prof Michael 68, 71, 81
omega fatty acids 41
osteoporosis 163
  African 163
  Maoris 164
overmass 156

P

palmitic acid, formula 40
pancreas cancer, alcohol 109
Parkinson's disease 47, 174
pastas, diet 128
percutaneous transluminal coronary angioplasty (PTCA) 73
pernicious anaemia 146
PGE1, effect on hypertension 136
  in thymus 144, 144f
pharmaceutical industry, powerhouse 86
pharmacy benefit management companies 86
Polynesians, genetic race 22
polyunsaturated fatty acids (PUFA) 52
  increases in 23
pre-eclampsia 166
premenstrual syndrome 166
progesterone, negative effect of statins 81
programmer, dietary 22
prostaglandins 41f, 134f, 157
  in diabetes 140
  in female disorders 166
  in hypertension 137
  in rheumatoid arthritis 143
prostate, benign hypertrophy 152
  cancer, smoking 106
  specific antigen (PSA) 152
PUFAs 145f
  in thymus 144, 145f
  cancer, animal experiments 149

R

races, results of intermingling 24
Recalled for Life (Sattilaro) 152

receptors 25f
Recommended Daily Averages 37t, 102, 103t
refining of foods, effects 32
  micronutrient loss 36
refrigeration, effects on food 89
relaxation 110
research, relative vs absolute statistics 71
respiratory system, prostaglandins 43, 44f
rheumatism 141
rheumatoid arthritis 47, 141
  criteria 142
Rhinehart and Greenberg, Drs, vitamin experiments 62
rice, in diet 127
risk factors, coronary, known, 74
  Hopkins and Williams 100
roller mills, introduction of 32, 58
Roman, ancient diets 121

S
salads, diet 121
salt, diet 127
sandwiches, diet 121
saturated fats 39
  does not increase cholesterol 97
Scandinavian Simvastin Survival Study (SSSS) 80
Scheepers, Dr Gunning 71
scleroderma 145
semen, decreased counts 166
seretonin 153, 153f, 166, 171
Seven Countries Study 48, 49, 49t, 59
  latest 1995 83
Seven Day Cure for RA 143
sex functions, prostaglandins 44f
Sinclair, Dr H.M. 46t
Sino-Japanese, diet 121
  genetic race 22
Sjogren's disease 145, 145f
smoking 105
  advice on stopping 107
  vs alcoholism 109
sorghum, basic food of Africans 37
  contents 116t, 117
  in hypertension 138
  in osteoporosis 164
  refining 37, 38f
soy protein 128
spastic colon 134, 146

spreads, diet 120
Stare, Olsen and Whelan, Drs 72
starvation 160
statins, cholesterol breakthrough 80
sterility 166
steroids, danger of prolonged use 146
  therapy for RA 142, 143
stress proteins 47
strokes 166
  homocysteine 78, 167
subterfuges for diet 129
Sudalipid, effect on blood cholesterol 97, 97t
sugar, diet 128
sunflower oil, fatty acid content 42
supplementation of micronutrients 115
surgery, heart 72
systemic lupus erythematosis (SLE) 47, 145, 145f, 146

T
Tactrine 169
tau protein 169
Taylor, Elizabeth, diet 159
testosterone, negative effects of statins 81
thrombophlebitis 167
thrombosis, venous 134f
thromboxanes 41f, 134f
thymus 144, 145f
time factor, new environmental factors 32
TIME, on CPPT trial 66
T-lymphocytes 145f
Tourette syndrome 173
triglycerides 60, 61f, 62
transfatty acids 45, 53
  bread 118
  elaidic acid 54
  International Life Sciences Institute 56
  vaccenic acid 54
tryptophane 154f, 166, 171
  dioxygenase 173
Tunstall-Pedoe, Dr 72
Two Centuries of American Medicine 31
tyrosine 154f

U
unsaturated fats 39
urticaria 145

uterus cancer 166

V
vegetables, in diet 126-127
vegetable fat, consumption USA 99f
  oils 122
venous thrombosis, deep 167
  role of homocysteine 78
Vikings, deaths due to diet 114
vitamins, in metabolism 35
  B6 41f, 42, 62, 63f
  B12 63f
  C 41f, 42
  D, negative effects of statins 81
  experiments, Rhinehart and Greenberg 62
  shortages, classical signs 33, 33f
Vorster, Prof Estie, eggs 120

W
Warfarin, in DVT 167
West of Scotland study 80
wheat germ, content 118, 118f
Willett, Dr W.C. 53
Willis's Case Book, Dr 153
World Health Organisation, on alcohol 108

X
Xanthomata 26
X-legs 171

Y
Yellowlees, Dr W.W., criticism of role of commerce 57
Yerushalmy, Dr, criticism of fat theory 60

Z
Zinc 41f, 42